# Exploring Your Unplanned Pregnancy

# Exploring Your Unplanned Pregnancy

*Single Motherhood, Adoption, and Abortion Questions and Resources*

JEFF DUFFEY MD

**Exploring Your Unplanned Pregnancy:** *Single Motherhood, Adoption, and Abortion Questions and Resources* by Jeff Duffey MD

Previously published under the pen name Tyne Traverson

Copyright © 2015 by Cairde, Karuna & Hedd Publishing, LLC

All rights reserved. No part of this book may be reproduced, distributed, or transmitted in any form or by any means, including photocopying, recording, or other electronic or mechanical methods, without the prior written permission of the publisher, except in the case of brief quotations embodied in critical reviews and certain other noncommercial uses permitted by copyright law. Write to Cairde, Karuna & Hedd Publishing, c/o Taylor English Duma LLP, 1600 Parkwood Circle, Suite 400, Atlanta, Georgia 30339

ExploringYourUnplannedPregnancy.com

Cover by Aaniyah Ahmed | 99designs
99designs.com/profiles/aaniyah

Interior design by Williams Writing, Editing & Design
www.williamswriting.com

Index written by Carol Roberts of Roberts Indexing Services
www.robertsindexing.com

First Edition 2015

ISBN 978-0-9862583-8-1
Library of Congress Control Number 2015931573

URLs are provided for informational purposes only and their mention should not be considered a recommendation. The author is not responsible for the content of these sites. See the disclaimer in chapter 1 for more details.

The author would like to thank all the professionals from various fields who have so graciously offered their time and expertise in helping the author with the writing and editing of this book. They have made a valuable contribution. The author dedicates this book to them.

# Contents

Preface **xiii**

Acknowledgments **xvii**

1     Laying the Groundwork    1
*This Is Your Decision*
*Reaching Out to Others*
*Avoiding Overload*
*Examining Your Values*
*Remembering Reassuring Beliefs*
*A Range of Feelings*
*Handling Self-Destructive Feelings*
*Taking the Long View*
*The Decision-Making Process*
*Perseverance*

2     Basic Questions About Single Motherhood    9
*You*
*The Biological Father*
*Your Child*
*Your Family*

3     Basic Questions About Adoption    13
*The Two-Parent Family*
*The Role of the Adoption Agency in Reflecting Your Wishes*
*Types of Adoptions*
*Expenses*

*The Adoptive Parents*
*Your Future Relationship with Your Child*
*Issues About the Legal Father, the Biological Father, and Your Other Children*
*Comparing Risks*

4 Basic Questions About Abortion  21
*Ethical Issues*
*An Avoidance-Avoidance Conflict*
*Timing*
*Your Child's Interest*
*Outside Pressure*
*Emotional Health*
*Missing Motherhood*
*Illegal Abortions*
*Miscarriage*
*Abortion Types*

5 Single Motherhood Resources  35
*Books and Book Lists*
*Some Costs of Single Motherhood*
*Comprehensive Websites with Leads to Many Resources*
*Financial Assistance, Food Assistance, and Grants*
*Money Management*
*Saving Money*
*Sharing*
*Bartering*
*Avoiding Paying Full Price*
*Avoiding Extra Expenses*
*Doing It Yourself*
*Thinking Creatively About Making Money*
*Taking Care of You*

*Preparing to Date Again*
*Helping Your Child Get More Fathering*
*Being Approachable*
*Getting More Education and Job Skills*

6 Adoption Resources  49
*An Overview*
*Adoption Agencies*
*Independent Adoptions*
*Adoption Law*
*Maternity Homes*
*Choosing an Adoptive Family*
*Adoption Scams*
*Teen Pregnancy*
*Contraception*

7 Abortion Resources  55
*Seeking Answers About Your Pregnancy*
*Determining How Far Along You Are*
*Medical Abortion*
*Surgical Abortion*
*Examples of Specific Provider Websites*
*Finding a Provider*
*Paying for the Abortion*
*The Fetal Pain Issue*
*The Emotional Effects Issue*
*Emotional Support After the Abortion*
*The Laws in Your State About Abortion*
*Contraception*

8 Conclusion  67

## APPENDIX

**A-1** The Biological Father    71
  *Passionate*
  *Permanent*
  *Partner-Ready*
  *Problem-Solving*
  *Parent-Material*
  *Productive*
  *Personable*
  *Protective*
  *Secrets*
  *Unhappily Married*
  *His Parents*
  *Inherited Diseases*
  *Your Husband Is Not the Biological Father*

**A-2** Supplementary Questions About Single Motherhood    77
  *The Joys of Single Motherhood*
  *Positive Alternatives to Having a Child*
  *Single Mothering Skills*
  *The Effect of Your Single Motherhood on Others*
  *Handling Stress*
  *Physical Health Concerns*
  *Finances*
  *Your Energy*

**A-3** Supplementary Questions About Adoption    85
  *Considering Different Perspectives*
  *Explaining Your Adoption Process to Others*
  *Selflessness*

*The Adoptive Process*
*Added Responsibilities*
*Anticipating Future Relationships*

**A-4** Supplementary Questions About Abortion  **89**
*Preconceived Ideas*
*Another Abortion*
*Rh Incompatibility*

From the Author  **91**

Bibliography  **93**

Index  **97**

# Preface

Single motherhood? Adoption? Abortion? When you have an unplanned pregnancy, these are the decisions you have to face. Making the right decision is hard. Use the information and essential questions this book raises to help you carefully think through all of your options. *It was written, not to make you decide a specific way, but to help you make the right decision for you and your situation.*

If you already know what you want to do about your pregnancy, reviewing the questions may confirm that you've made the right decision for you. The practical information in the resource chapters will streamline your search for qualified assistance and save you time.

Your decision about your pregnancy is essentially irreversible at some point. You have to live with it the rest of your life. Can you afford not to study this book to make your decision your own well-thought-out selection?

In examining the drawbacks of each decision, you may start to feel as if any decision you make will be the wrong one. Women have decided on each of these options and years later been satisfied their decision was right for them. *You can make a decision that will be right for you as well.*

This book addresses your concerns whether you are married, in a relationship, or completely single. The term "single motherhood" is used in the title to underscore the fact that any woman may become a single mother. Through divorce, widowhood, the breakup of your relationship, or the health limitations of the biological father, you eventually may have to raise the child as a single mother.

Many women find that their perspectives on their pregnancy change over time. This change of perspectives is normal. It's important to consider everything you can: thoughts, feelings, plans, family, friends, culture, personal situations, values, and anything else that affects your decision.

This book appeared under the pen name Tyne Traverson until the author realized readers don't trust authors they can't know. Though the author is an MD, the important thing is whether what the author has written rings true to you.

This book attempts to be completely unbiased. Because certain words and phrases have so many negative or positive associations, using them can influence conclusions. Emotionally charged words like "pro-choice" or "pro-life" have been deliberately avoided. The purpose here is to help you make the best decision for you, whatever it is.

Women become pregnant under many circumstances. Your romantic partner and the sexual partner who is responsible for your pregnancy may not be the same person. For simplicity, this book will assume they are the same person and male. Even though your pregnancy may not result in their becoming a father, this person will be referred to as the "biological father" for consistency.

Adoptive parents are referred to as though they are male and female, though adoptive parents may be of the same sex or transgendered.

The phrase "placed for adoption" is used whether or not giving up the baby is a desired option. Sometimes a woman is in a situation that will not allow her to keep her baby even though she may want to. Although your situation is unique, it is hoped that you will feel a connection with the many women who have faced the same options that you face now.

Please study the book's table of contents. The first chapter lays the groundwork, then three chapters pose basic questions about each pregnancy decision. The next three chapters (5, 6, 7) each have resources depending on which decision you reach about your pregnancy. After a concluding chapter, an appendix provides additional resources. If you are considering being a single mother, then the chapter on the biological father and the supplementary chapter on single motherhood in the appendix will be helpful. If you are considering adoption or abortion, then the added information in those supplementary chapters will be useful.

## Disclaimer

Deciding what to do about an unplanned pregnancy is a complicated process. While the author expects this book can help you think about many of the issues involved, everyone has unique experiences that affect how they react. Even though the author hopes you do not have any problems from reading this book, the author takes no responsibility for how this book affects you. The author takes no responsibility for any decisions that you may make after reading it. Read this book at your own risk. Please question everything you read in this book. Ask yourself if the things written here ring true to your own experiences and beliefs.

Although the author and publisher of this book have made every effort to ensure the accuracy and completeness of this book, they cannot guarantee or warrant that the contents are accurate or complete. They also cannot be responsible for any of the third-party resources discussed in this book.

The information provided in this book is intended to help

you make an informed decision about what is best for you. It is not a substitute for medical advice or treatment. The author cannot give you medical advice and urges you to consult your physician before making any decisions regarding your pregnancy or any other health-related matters. Of course, you should feel free to discuss anything you read in this book with your physician.

Similarly, the information provided in this book is not a substitute for legal advice from a licensed attorney, and you should not consider anything in the book a solicitation of legal advice. If you have any legal questions or concerns, you should consult an attorney who is licensed in your state.

# Acknowledgments

The author could not have written this book without the help of many people. Their deep concern for you, the pregnant woman facing a difficult decision, went into the work of writing this book.

The author wishes to acknowledge the profound contribution made by this book's developmental editor, whose wisdom, thoroughness, and loving concern helped make it what it is.

# 1

## *Laying the Groundwork*

### This Is Your Decision

Opinions and advice are given in some parts of this book. These opinions and advice, however, are not about which decision you should make about your pregnancy. This is no accident. This book was written to help you think about your decision thoroughly. It was not written to make you decide a specific way. It is not the purpose of this book to lead you to make a particular decision.

There is risk in any decision-making process, but a decision about your pregnancy requires you to face some difficult consequences. Each decision has varying degrees of social disapproval associated with it. Each is essentially irreversible at some point. You will have to live with this decision for the rest of your life, so make it your own decision. Don't allow anyone to take the decision away from you. Think for yourself. Read this book with an open mind. By thinking about it thoroughly now, you will be able to say to yourself later that you honestly gave every possibility a fair hearing.

Perhaps your experiences and life situation make your decision obvious to you. Reading this book could confirm your decision.

This book won't just help you think through your decision, it will also help you follow through with your decision by providing connections to resources and people who can help you.

## Reaching Out to Others

Use this book as a beginning, not an ending, to your decision-making process. Use it as one part of a larger conversation with people important in your life.

It might be easier to start by talking with someone not directly affected by your situation, like an OB/GYN or family physician. Gynecology is the study of the treatment of women's diseases. Obstetrics is the study of the treatment of pregnancy, birth, and the postpartum period. All physicians specializing in these fields are trained in both fields and are called OB/GYNs. OB/GYNs have experience helping women. Perhaps you already have an OB/GYN or family physician you can count on to listen to you, accept you, and help you in making your own decision.

Do you know someone who has been through this situation? Are there coaches or teachers in your life who put you at ease because they are so accepting of you? Are there grandparents whose eyes have always lit up when they saw you? Perhaps a religious person who has known you all your life could be your wise listener. What about your roommate?

Could you start with the member of your family or your biological father's family most likely to be open and helpful? Are you ready to talk with your biological father? Some people start the talking process with God.

To start these discussions, you could share this book with a trusted person in your life.

## Avoiding Overload

Women of all ages and backgrounds may find this book useful, but if you find it is too difficult to read for any reason, share this book with someone else you trust. Let him or her select what parts of it to discuss with you. You can then talk about it in smaller steps. It is good to know your limitations.

## Examining Your Values

Making a decision requires examining your values. Every woman has her own set of experiences and religious or ethical beliefs that help shape her values and influence her decision.

Different women may decide that any one of the three pregnancy decisions is the most loving one for them in their particular situation. They may think that their particular decision is in the best interest of everyone involved.

For example, one woman may decide to make sacrifices and raise her child alone because she thinks she can do it well. Another woman is willing to have an abortion because she thinks ending the pregnancy is better than subjecting her child to a difficult life. A third woman decides on adoption and gives her child the gift of a two-parent family.

## Remembering Reassuring Beliefs

As you read this book, remembering the beliefs you already hold may be reassuring. For example, do you believe God is like a loving parent who does not want you to make mistakes, who still loves you when you do, who offers you forgiveness when you ask, and who accepts you as you are? If you believe that, then do you think God could also forgive you if you made the mistake of being a single mother, made the mistake of placing your child up for adoption, or made the mistake of having an abortion?

## A Range of Feelings

You may think there is something wrong with you because of the conflicted feelings you have about your pregnancy. Other women can tell you that it is human and natural to have a whole range of feelings now. You may be feeling bewildered by the confusing mixture of strong emotions. It may help you to try to identify some of these feelings.

What will you do with these feelings? Can you accept that, at least for now, this is how you feel? Some feelings may change and some may not. Do not ignore them. Talk about them with people you trust. Realize that others have felt the same feelings and have still found a way to make decisions and succeed.

If you are happy, that's wonderful. If you are not happy, realize that things can change and that you can be part of making those changes.

## Handling Self-Destructive Feelings

If you are feeling self-destructive, then it is urgent that you talk with someone who can help you *now*. If you cannot think of anyone to call, call 911 and tell them how you are feeling. The National Suicide Hotline is available 24/7 at 1–800–273–8255. You can also go to a hospital emergency room.

After you have gotten immediate help, learn ways to deal with future suicidal thoughts by working with a counselor. Talk with your family doctor about whether you might have depression and might benefit from medication. Consider reading Thomas Ellis and Cory Newman's book *Choosing to Live: How to Defeat Suicide Through Cognitive Therapy*.

## Taking the Long View

When you think about dealing with your feelings about the pregnancy, examine your strengths. Are you physically healthy? Are you young and do you have many more years of life before you? What are some life problems you have already overcome? What are the things you have already done in your life? What are the skills that you have already learned? Parenting is a set of skills that gets better with practice, like playing a sport or driving a car.

Did you ever think something in your life was never going to get better or change, but it somehow did? How can you be so sure that nothing is going to get better about your pregnancy? Is it possible that you're underestimating how loved and accepted you are by your parents, friends, and family? Is it possible you're not giving them the benefit of the doubt? Could talking about this pregnancy be an opportunity for them to show you how much they accept and believe in you when even you find it difficult to believe in you?

It can feel as if your world stopped when you realized that you were pregnant, but it is important to see your pregnancy in a broader view. While it is a serious situation and deserves your best thinking, it is not the end of your life. You may not be able to believe it now, but there will be times when you will laugh again, when a sunrise will again move you to wonder, when you will have a sense of belonging, when you will feel more like you, and life will feel more manageable. Time will help. Take the long view.

## The Decision-Making Process

Not all the elements in your decision are of equal importance. Some questions simply will not apply to you. Your situation may differ from someone else's. What might be very important to her may not be important to you. Could it be possible that what might be right for you once, may not be right for you at another time if you or your situation changes?

In making decisions, it is sometimes possible to be blindsided by something that you may have overlooked, have never experienced, or did not fully appreciate. Because of this, it can be very helpful to gather as much information as possible and to have help from others in making decisions.

Some questions concern problems that you may face. When you get to these questions, you'll want to ask yourself whether you could solve the problem later by learning something new, practicing a skill, making a change in you, or getting help from others.

Wanting to do something is different from needing to do something. Most women don't intentionally get pregnant because they "want" to have an abortion or be a single mother. Most women would not say that they got pregnant because they wanted to place their child with an adoptive family. Therefore, when you pick one of these three possibilities, it is because you need to pick it, because you think it is the best of the three, and not because you intentionally wanted to have to make that decision.

Another thing about the decisions is that they do not all have to be made at once, but some decisions are made for you if you wait too long. Specific types of abortions are done only at specific times in the pregnancy. At some point in the pregnancy, the law does not allow abortion unless there are medical reasons for it.

Although it is possible to decide to place your child for adoption after it is born, it would be much easier to start the process before that time and have some of your expenses paid.

If you do nothing, you will be a single mother by not taking any action. That might be the best decision for you, but if it is made just because you do nothing, you may regret your passivity. When the women who have picked abortion or adoption have gone through with their decisions, as a single mother your multiyear responsibility will just be beginning. You will not be able to remain passive and be an effective single mother.

## Perseverance

Sometimes you are in a situation in which you cannot get an abortion or cannot place your child with an adoptive family, and you find yourself having to be a single mother. The questions in the chapter on single motherhood have to do with the positives and negatives of being a single mother.

If you must be a single mother, do not despair. Other women have done it and found that things that seemed insurmountable could often be overcome in time with others' help, with opportunities that they did not have at first, and with their personal growth. It may be difficult, but it is possible. Think about the women you know who are widowed or divorced, and who raised their children successfully.

Many women feel unprepared at first to raise a child. Having a single mother may not be as good for a child as having two parents, but single-mothered children do cope and do thrive. Do not give up hope. You are not alone. If you believe God cares about you, then be mindful of that.

This book makes some assumptions about your freedom to decide, and perhaps your situation does not allow that freedom. Have courage. Things can change. If you already know that you are going to be a single mother, then you can use the single motherhood chapter to look at the challenges that you will be dealing with. Use the resource chapter to find some specifics about how to deal with those challenges.

# 2

## *Basic Questions About Single Motherhood*

Not all these questions will apply to you. This book tries to reach a variety of people: people of various ages and education, and people with many situations. As you review these questions, remember that there are resources in later chapters that can help you with answering them.

### You

Immediately after learning that you were pregnant, what was your first feeling/thought/gut response?

If you learned that your first pregnancy test was incorrect and the more accurate repeat test showed you were not pregnant, how would you feel? Does that say anything about your wishes?

You may be very capable of being a mother and yet know in your heart that motherhood is not for you. There is nothing wrong with you. Can you satisfy your need to nurture others in another way?

Is being a parent the life you want?

Do you want a baby?

## The Biological Father

Are you and the biological father in love?

Is the biological father a responsible, loving, kind person who loves you and makes you a priority?

Is it best to have the baby now and with the partner you have?

Would the biological father make a good parent and provider for your child if you decided to have one?

Raising a child involves solving problems. Does the biological father work well with you in solving problems?

Even if you answered yes to these questions, you may want to read chapter A-1 in the appendix entitled "The Biological Father." That chapter deals with the biological father, your relationship, and the personal qualities the biological father should have to be a good parent. Because these personal qualities are required for you to be a good parent, you can use the chapter's questions to assess your readiness as well.

## Your Child

Do you already have experience with children and skills at taking care of them?

A child will count on you to have all of his or her needs met. A child will count on you, and will never stop counting on you, day after day after day. You are your child's final safety net. Are you ready for that responsibility? Can you become ready for that responsibility? (Chapter 5, "Single Motherhood Resources," lists some help available to you to meet these responsibilities.)

Can you afford to have a baby? (You may want to look at chapter 5, "Single Motherhood Resources," and follow the links to the websites where you can determine how much it costs to have a baby.)

If it would be financially difficult to raise a baby, have you grown up in situations of hardship such that you already know how to manage money and cope with not having enough of it?

## Your Family

How would the children you might have later be affected by your having this child now?

Would having a baby now interfere with your ability to care for your existing children and other family members? How will your other children and partner feel about their having to share even less of your limited time, money, and energy?

Are you compromising the biological father's future by having a baby? Your future? Your parents' future? Could having a baby now brighten everyone's future? Is your mother excited to be a grandmother? Is the biological father's mother excited to be a grandmother? Do they seem more excited about it than you do? You aren't having a baby for them, are you?

Do your parents tell you about any health problems that they have? Do they have any chronic illnesses that could make it difficult for them to help you? For example, does either of them have low back pain that would make it difficult to lift a baby? Is their health good enough for them to have the energy they need to help you?

Is it fair to ask your family members to sacrifice their time, energy, money, and life plans so you do not have to raise your child alone, so you don't have to place your child in an adoptive family, or so you don't have to have an abortion?

After you have read this chapter and the resources chapter, if you feel as though you need more information about single motherhood, chapter A-2, "Supplementary Questions About Single Motherhood," in the appendix provides a more thorough look at being a single parent. It may help you consider things you have not yet thought of. You will be clearer about your decision and more prepared to act on it if you read the supplementary chapter.

# 3

## *Basic Questions About Adoption*

This chapter will first ask you to consider the advantages of adoption for your child. Then it will use questions to outline practical aspects of adoption such as expenses, legal issues, the adoption agency, adoptive parents, health risks, and your future relationship with your child.

What are your preconceived notions about adoption and the women who place their child with an adoptive family?

## The Two-Parent Family

Adoption has the benefit of giving your child two chosen adoptive parents who live together in one home. Sometimes that second person is a father. Admittedly, some fathers are better than others are. It is not simply having a man around, but having a good man around, that benefits your child.

In the author's opinion, in an ideal situation, having a father living at home with him can give a boy a chance to learn how to be a father himself one day. A boy sees how his own father acts with him and how his own father copes with life each day. A boy learns by imitating his dad. A boy observes how his father shows his love to his mother each day in various situations. A boy notices how his mother and father solve problems as partners. Some of his own identity and self-worth comes from being his father's son.

Fathers do things differently than mothers. They give a child a sense that the child isn't so fragile. They roughhouse some. Fathers are more hands-on. They illustrate hardiness. They introduce the child to the world of things. Sometimes fathers emphasize performance when mothers are accepting regardless. Their expectations can be a vote of confidence to the child. They give children a sense of what they should do. This allows moms to be more unconditionally accepting and provides a balance between thoughts and feelings. Sometimes parents change roles and the child gets to see flexibility as well.

The twinkle a father has in his eye when he sees his daughter is valuable to her sense of feeling loved and accepted for being herself. Her relationship with her father is an opportunity to practice being feminine in an atmosphere of safety and acceptance. A girl sees the model of how her mother relates to her father and how they successfully solve disagreements while continuing to support each other as people. Having a father in the home gives a girl an opportunity to learn to share because she has to share her father with her mother. As a girl grows up and must start to detach from her mother somewhat, she can find some security in having an ally in her dad.

Not only does an adopted child gain a father, the child benefits from having a mother refreshed and emotionally supported by that father. A father's help makes it easier for the adoptive mother to be effective because she has more sleep, more money, and more time. Having a father around allows the adoptive mother to take a break. A father solves the problem of who will care for her child if she cannot.

Many of these advantages apply to children with adoptive parents from gay and lesbian partnerships as well. You may know gay and lesbian parents who make a point of providing their adopted children with frequent chances to be with role models of the opposite sex from the parents.

## The Role of the Adoption Agency in Reflecting Your Wishes

Do you realize that in an open adoption you can provide information about you and your family's health and other history, know biographical information about adoptive parents, and have a say in who becomes your child's adoptive parents? Do you know that, by picking your adoption agency and your adoption type, you can have some say in how much is known about you and how much you know about the adoptive family? Do you know that you can meet them?

Do you know that in some agencies you can pick whether or not you want the adoptive parents by your bedside for the birth? Do you know you can decide whether you want time alone with your baby, or you can decide not to see your baby at all?

Laws regulate adoption agencies. Some adoption agencies belong to organizations that agree to honor additional specific standards. Do you think you can satisfy yourself that you have an excellent adoption agency by using the Internet and making phone calls to check?

Are you in a state that requires a brief foster home placement before final adoption?

## Types of Adoptions

Do you want an open adoption where the child knows you, corresponds with you, and so on? Do you want a closed adoption where you have the most privacy and the child cannot find you? Do you want something in between? (See "Adoption

Resources," chapter 6, for links to more details about your options.)

Do you know the advantages and disadvantages of having an independent adoption through a doctor or lawyer? (See chapter 6, "Adoption Resources.")

If you opt for a private adoption, your doctor or lawyer will find an adoptive couple. You may also look for an adoptive family among people you know. Could any of these people adopt your child: mother, father, sister, brother, aunt, cousin, coworker, teacher, neighbor, or member of your religious group?

## Expenses

The adoptive parents may pay for some legally determined pregnancy-related expenses, depending on what you work out with them or the adoption agency. Some of these expenses could include prenatal visits, vitamins, hospital bills, surgical bills, sonograms, and other costs directly related to your pregnancy. Will you find a way to pay for these expenses otherwise?

Will you be able to work during your pregnancy?

Will continuing your pregnancy so you can place your baby with an adoptive family require you to drop out of school for a time or take Internet courses?

In the past, pregnant women would leave their town and go to a home for unwed mothers to hide their pregnancies and be able to arrange an adoption in secret. Things have changed some since those times, but this could still be a good decision for some women. Do you have a situation now that makes others knowing about your pregnancy unthinkable and requires going away? Can you live with a relative in another town to save expenses? Some adoption agencies will pay for housing or have special maternity housing. Do you know of a maternity home in a not too distant area? (See chapter 6, "Adoption Resources.")

## The Adoptive Parents

Have you considered how you can minimize your worry about how qualified the adoptive parents will be? (See chapter 6, "Adoption Resources," to learn about thoroughly investigating your adoption agency's procedures.)

Do you know it is possible to make sure your contract with the adoption agency and adoptive parents has a provision that the adoptive parents will not back out if your child has special needs?

In an open adoption, are you willing to pursue getting enough information about the adoptive parents to assure you that they will allow you to know how your child is doing and make it possible for you to have a connection with your child? Do you think it is important to choose a couple who can respect what you have done for them? Do you think you are a good-enough judge of character to ensure that the adopting couple can relate to you well in the future? How do you see the biological father interacting with the adoptive parents?

Check out the adoption resources to see that, as part of the selection process, adoptive parents are expected to talk frankly about themselves and their values.

## Your Future Relationship with Your Child

Even your children who live with you can blame you for things over which you have no control. They can go through times of rejecting you, can be rebellious, can get jealous of your other children, can play people against each together, can withhold affection, and can fail to understand what you are doing for them.

Do you think you can weather the difficulties of relating to your child through the filter of adoption? Adopted children are likely to be happy and have positive feelings about their adoption and the birthmother. The resources in chapter 6 discuss this issue.

## Issues About the Legal Father, the Biological Father, and Your Other Children

If you are married, how would your husband feel about giving up parental rights?

In many states, if you are a married woman who wants to place a child with an adoptive family, your husband, as the "legal father," must agree. The "legal father" often has more significant legal rights than the "biological father." Different states vary on how they determine whether a man who has lived with you can be considered the "legal father."

If you became pregnant by your husband and then later divorce, different states will treat that situation differently. In addition, if you are married and become pregnant by someone other than your husband, your husband can still refuse to allow the child to be placed with an adoptive family. If you are in one of these situations, it is very important that you contact a lawyer familiar with adoption laws in your state.

If you wait too long to learn the legal issues related to adoption for your case, your other options will be more limited. If your husband is abusive or unstable, a lawyer may also help you determine whether the court could take away his parental rights.

If you decide to keep the adoption secret, do you feel you can tolerate the risk of your secret later being revealed to your new partner and new kids?

How would going through a pregnancy now affect your relationships with those around you? Could you still fulfill your responsibilities to them?

Will you be able to have another child later? Are you nearing the end of your childbearing years?

## Comparing Risks

It is important to consider the risks involved in your pregancy. Whether you decide to keep the baby or whether you place the baby for adoption, you will go through labor and delivery just the same. Your risks of giving birth are no different whether you adopt or keep the baby.

If you go through a pregnancy, you will have the risks of pregnancy, of labor, and of delivery. You will have the risk of birth complications, bleeding, blood clots, and preeclampsia. Preeclampsia is a condition that can result in high blood pressure, swelling, protein in the mother's urine, and damage to the lining of blood vessels. It must be treated to avoid seizures and the risk of death. Sometimes it may require a premature termination of the pregnancy to save the mother's life. The resources chapters can help you consider these risks. Do you know about the risks already?

Your doctor may decide that a Caesarian section, often called a C-section, would be the best way for you to give birth. A C-section is a surgical procedure in which the surgeon makes an incision in the woman's abdominal wall and uterus to remove the baby. It is performed on an emergency basis when the baby is in distress during labor or there is difficulty with the baby moving through the birth canal. It is used on a planned basis for a variety of reasons, such as when it is already known that the shape and size of a woman's pelvic bones give her a small outlet and the baby has a big head.

If you have an abortion, you will go through a different procedure with different risks. The earlier you have the abortion, the less your risk. From a statistical point of view, abortion procedures done early in the pregnancy have less risk than giving birth. You will want to research the exact figures using the resource chapters. Late gestation abortions have potential for greater risk than normal births.

When you read "Adoption Resources," chapter 6, you will learn that there are professionals available to help you at each step of the adoption process. You may be surprised that adoption today is not what you thought it was, and the worries you had about it were based on the way adoption used to be or the stereotypes you saw in movies and books. The questions in chapter A-3, "Supplementary Questions About Adoption," touch on long-term concerns related to adoption.

# 4

## *Basic Questions About Abortion*

This chapter discusses different aspects of abortion, describes the types of abortions, and explains miscarriage.

The questions in the "Ethical Issues" section below are some of the most important ones in this book. They are also some of the most difficult and potentially overwhelming questions.

If you feel you might become overwhelmed, skim through the "Ethical Issues" questions without trying to answer them now. Read the educational information in the rest of this chapter. Read each resource chapter. You will be better informed and will discover there are helpful people and resources available for each decision path. Having this background will help you feel more equipped to take on the "Ethical Issues" questions. Additionally, your brain will have been unconsciously processing the questions since you first read them. When you come back to these important "Ethical Issues" questions, consider working through them with someone you trust.

### Ethical Issues

It is not the purpose of this book to tell you what to believe about abortion. The views of different people are offered here to give you more information to help you make your own decision. There are too many views to include them all.

Instead, this book presents views across the full spectrum without endorsing any particular view.

Some people believe abortion is morally wrong under any circumstances and that abortion is murder. Others believe abortion ordinarily is morally wrong but may be necessary in certain circumstances, such as in the case of needing to save the life of the mother, of rape, of incest, or when the child would be born with serious birth defects.

Some people believe abortion is justified because the greater wrong is forcing a child to live in a situation in which he or she will have a hard life. Some children are born into extreme poverty and other clearly unlivable conditions. Some people believe abortion is justified because these children have a right to a good life or the right to have no life at all. Some people believe if you cannot give a child a good life at the time of your pregnancy, then you do not have the right to have a child then. They believe having a child in these circumstances is morally wrong and cruel. It is not this book's purpose to tell you when life begins or whether you should believe in the right of a child to have a good life or not have to live one at all. These questions are designed to help you explore your own values, thoughts, and feelings about these issues.

What kind of life is possible for a child you would have at this time?

How hard does your child's life have to be before you can allow him or her not to have to live it?

Some people believe a woman has the right to decide what to do with her body, regardless of her situation, because it is her body. Some people see adoption as preferable to abortion, and others do not.

There are also many opinions about when life begins. Some people believe life begins at conception. Some believe at first there is just a clump of developing cells then an embryo. *Embryo* is a term generally used to describe the human organism in the first full eight weeks of pregnancy. After the end of the eighth week, the term *fetus* is generally used. Some people believe life begins with the fetal heartbeat or fetal movement. Some people believe the fetus does not become a baby until it is born.

At some point, the government determines what constitutes viability (when the fetus can live on its own outside the mother's body) and the government will not allow abortions beyond that point.

What you believe about when life begins may have a bearing on whether you think abortion can be a moral decision. It may also have a bearing on whether you believe abortions at some points in the pregnancy are okay and others, done later, are not.

According to your particular religious beliefs, what are the religious consequences of having an abortion? Are the consequences the same regardless of when or why you had the abortion? Do you believe you can be forgiven if you do something that your religion believes is wrong?

If you believe in prayer, can you talk to God about your unplanned pregnancy?

How clear-cut do you believe God is about abortion? Does God have different rules for different situations or is there just one rule for all situations? Do you believe God would forgive you for having an abortion?

Do you believe that God would forgive you if you brought a child into the world by mistake and later realized that the child was going to have a miserable life?

If you are a religious person, consider whether talking to a person important in your religious life would help in coming to an understanding of these issues. Whether or not you are religious, finding a thoughtful person who will be open-minded as they listen to you think this through might be helpful.

## An Avoidance-Avoidance Conflict

There are different types of conflict situations. When you go to an ice cream store, you have an approach-approach conflict because you must pick just one flavor out of several you might want.

If you have to pick between eating ice cream and gaining weight from eating it, you have an approach-avoidance conflict. You would like to have the ice cream but avoid the weight gain.

Whether to have an abortion is an avoidance-avoidance conflict. You may want to avoid having an abortion, but you may also want to avoid single motherhood or adoption.

A woman gets an abortion because she feels the consequences of not getting one are clearly worse than the consequences of getting one. In your particular situation now, what are the specific consequences, if any, that come to your mind?

As you were reading the chapters on single motherhood and adoption, what did you find you most wanted to avoid happening, if anything, by having an abortion?

## Timing

Raising a child is hard work. Things have to be done when the child needs them to be done, not on the mother's schedule. Having an abortion allows you to put this off until you are in a better position to do it well. Is this a good time to have your child?

Having an abortion allows you to pick being childless as well.

## Your Child's Interest

While having an abortion avoids the mental distress associated with single motherhood, more importantly, it may allow a child to avoid needlessly living a hard life. If you believe you are keeping a child from living a hard life, do you also believe that you have your child's interest at heart when you pick abortion?

Single mothers and women who pick adoption make sacrifices for what they think is best for their children. They risk being ridiculed, misunderstood, and condemned by others. Is a woman who decides to have an abortion so her child does not have to live a hard life making a sacrifice too? Could this sacrifice be in the best interest of her child?

Is it possible that all the women who make each of these decisions could be making these sacrifices out of love for their children, born or never born?

## Outside Pressure

Is one advantage of having an abortion that it would be what the biological father or your family wants you to do?

Do you feel forced into having an abortion when you don't want one?

Do you feel forced into not having an abortion when you do want one?

## Emotional Health

As you read these questions, remember there is more information about these issues in "Abortion Resources," chapter 7.

An abortion is quick compared with a nine-month pregnancy. It is much quicker than eighteen-plus years of raising a child. How long do you think it will take you to readjust emotionally from the experience of having an abortion? Are you basing your estimate on what you have heard in the media or do you know the research about it? (See "Abortion Resources," chapter 7, for more information.) How long do you think it will it take the biological father to mentally process the abortion?

What is the current state of your mental health? This question is a very important one to consider. Women already having problems with their mental health may have a harder time dealing with having an abortion. Which would be hardest on you mentally—dealing with having had an abortion, placing your child with an adoptive family, or raising a child yourself?

If you were forced not to have an abortion, how would you feel about having to raise an unwanted child? Do you think it would affect your ability to form a bond with that child?

## Missing Motherhood

If you get an abortion, will you later feel you have missed the pleasures of motherhood? These pleasures might include watching your child grow up and discover the world, having a sense of being part of the cycle of life, having a chance to teach and shape someone, and having the love of a child who may adore you. Is this your last chance to have children?

## Illegal Abortions

As laws change, making it harder to get an abortion in some cities and states, women seeking abortions may feel they have no other option but to turn to a person providing abortions illegally. Under these conditions, there are no regulations or inspections to determine the skills of the provider, the sterility of the operation site, the adequacy of the equipment, and the competence of the assisting staff. What would ordinarily be a low-risk surgical procedure then becomes one potentially much more risky.

If you attempt to cause your own abortion by inserting something up your vagina, you could accidentally stick the instrument through the wall of your uterus and bleed to death or cause a serious infection. An unskilled abortion provider could do the same thing to you.

If a woman develops an infection after an illegal abortion, there may not be any follow-up care provided. This lack of treatment could become very serious. If the infection leads to shock from a massive infection getting into her bloodstream, the woman might die.

The umbilical cord runs from the fetus to the placenta. The placenta is a flat structure attached to the wall of the uterus. Nourishment goes through the placenta to the fetus. Waste products from the fetus go through the placenta to the mother. The placenta also produces hormones to support the pregnancy.

If the placenta is not completely removed from the lining of the uterus during the abortion, the uterus will "think" that the woman is still pregnant, and the uterine blood vessels will still be dilated and bleeding. This is a medical emergency. If the woman does not quickly have a D&C (dilation and curettage) for this incomplete abortion, she will continue to bleed, putting her life at great risk. (In performing a D&C, a surgeon first causes the cervical opening to enlarge and become wider. Then the surgeon uses an instrument with a small loop at the end, a curette, to gently scrape the inside surface of the uterus.)

If any problem with the illegal abortion develops, the woman may delay going to an emergency room because she doesn't want to get herself or others in trouble. She could bleed to death, possibly in her sleep. Please don't get an illegal abortion—it is too risky.

Unfortunately, the presence of unskilled providers offering illegal abortions makes the public mistakenly believe all abortions are dangerous. In "Abortion Resources," chapter 7, you will find links to websites that will spell out under what conditions having an abortion actually is less risky than having a baby.

## Miscarriage

A similar problem with bleeding can happen to a pregnant woman who miscarries. Such a miscarriage is called a *spontaneous abortion* to distinguish it from an *elective therapeutic abortion*, which is planned and thus not spontaneous. It is not uncommon for women to miscarry. Even though a woman wants a baby, she may be unable to carry it to term. If the lining of the uterus is not shed properly in a miscarriage, the woman will also bleed and will need a dilation and curettage procedure to stop the bleeding. If this should happen to you and you cannot immediately reach your doctor, go the emergency room.

Sometimes a woman may mistakenly believe her mixed feelings about the pregnancy resulted in a miscarriage. You cannot think yourself into miscarrying. On the other hand, if you are waiting to see if you miscarry in hopes that your pregnancy decision will solve itself, your delay may prevent you from getting an abortion early and make your surgical risks go up if you decide to have an abortion later.

## Abortion Types

You may find it helpful to have some terms defined as this discussion moves from talking about abortion as an abstract concept to talking about it as a clinical procedure.

Sometimes an abortion is performed for medical reasons—because the mother's life is at risk otherwise. When an abortion isn't performed for medical reasons, it's called an *elective abortion*.

States vary in when they will allow women to have elective abortions, and these laws sometimes change, so it's important to learn what the current laws are in your state. Some states will not allow an elective abortion after twenty weeks, and other states will not allow an elective abortion after twenty-four weeks. Laws in different states describe the kinds of situations in which exceptions can be made after that time. For example, in one state an exception might be made if the continuation of the pregnancy endangers the mother's life. Another state may grant an exception if the continuation of the pregnancy endangers the mother's health.

The websites listed in chapter 7, "Abortion Resources," contain details about the different types of abortions and walk you through the different steps. Some websites will help you compare the different types of abortions.

You may see the word *gestation* used to talk about pregnancy. Gestation is the period of development of the human organism in the uterus from the time of conception until birth. In short, it is the pregnancy. If you were entering your thirty-sixth week of pregnancy, you would say you were at thirty-six weeks' gestation.

**Medical Abortions.** A medicine is used to cause the abortion. A pregnant woman's body produces a lot of progesterone. This hormone keeps the uterine lining thick and the pregnancy implanted in the uterus. A medicine called mifepristone, or RU-486, blocks progesterone. If a woman takes RU-486, over days (or rarely, weeks) the uterine lining thins enough that the pregnancy detaches. Another medicine, misoprostol, is taken within a few days of the mifepristone and it causes the uterus to contract. Usually in the next day, the woman then has what looks like a heavy period with blood clots and some pregnancy tissue. Another variation of this uses methotrexate, a medication that stops the ongoing implantation process of the pregnancy. After taking methotrexate for several days, the pregnant woman then takes misoprostol to cause the uterus to contract with the same results as with mifepristone.

These procedures are most effective in the first seven weeks of pregnancy, but have been used up to the first 70 days. Some women who have a medical abortion find that it is not effective in terminating the pregnancy, and then go on to have a surgical abortion. A medical abortion requires several visits to the doctor.

**Surgical Abortions.** In these surgeries, the pregnancy is terminated by removing the embryo or fetus from the uterus. You must wait about seven weeks before having any surgical abortion because the embryo is too small to be found before that time. The surgical tool would miss the embryo and the pregnancy would continue unaffected. Doctors doing surgical abortions may use pain medicines, antianxiety medicines, sedation, numbing medication, or anesthesia, depending on the situation. The following types of abortion are all surgical abortions. Medical and other considerations may extend or shorten the time frame in which a particular surgical abortion can be done. These suggested surgical time frames are approximate.

**Manual Vacuum Aspiration (MVA).** This type of abortion is usually done between seven and nine weeks of pregnancy. The doctor uses a gentle handheld tool, called an aspirator, which uses suction to remove the lining of the uterus and the implanted embryo. Remember that you lose the lining of your uterus every month when you have an ordinary menstrual period.

**Standard Vacuum Aspiration.** This type of abortion is generally done usually between seven and fourteen weeks of pregnancy (in some places sixteen weeks of pregnancy) and involves using another suction apparatus to vacuum out the lining of the uterus. The procedure takes a few minutes, and some medical centers will confirm that the abortion has been effective before you leave the center.

**Dilation and Evacuation (D&E).** This type of abortion is usually performed if it has been seven to sixteen weeks *since a woman's last menses.* More than one visit may be required. It may be necessary for a woman's cervix dilation to be started the night before the procedure is completed. (To understand the cervix, imagine the uterus is an upside-down pear. At the lower part of the upside-down pear is the neck of the pear. The neck of the pear corresponds to the cervix. The cervix has an opening where the stem would be. That opening is the entrance to the uterus. It can be gently enlarged (or *dilated*) if need be.

The D&E procedure takes longer than the Standard Vacuum Aspiration and involves removing the contents of the uterus with suction or a surgical instrument. The fetal heart is stopped quickly by an injection of potassium or a heart drug that does not harm the mother. It has been written that the fetus's nervous system is not well-developed enough to feel pain. The procedure should be done by a provider who does the procedure often enough to be experienced and do it well.

Ask your provider about his or her experience. Don't hesitate to ask about your particular situation and how it affects your risk. Healthcare providers are your best source of information because they know your particular situation, and risk can vary with the situation. It may be less or more than you think.

On unusual occasions, abortion procedures done late in the pregnancy can have surgical risks significantly greater than giving birth; on other occasions, the risk may not be as high as childbirth.

**Saline-Induced Abortion.** Saline is water that has a specific amount of salt in it. This technique involves injecting a saltwater solution into the amniotic sac (the fluid-filled sac surrounding the embryo), which causes labor and delivery over a period of hours. Other variations on this procedure involve injecting substances other than saltwater. Some stories you may have heard from older women about abortions have to do with this type of abortion, which required going into labor.

This abortion technique has been replaced almost completely by the D&E-type abortion, which has a lower rate of complications when done by a skilled provider. Rarely, providers who have not acquired the new skills to do D&Es use saline-induced abortion.

## 4: Basic Questions About Abortion

The websites listed in chapter 7, "Abortion Resources," contain details about the different types of abortions and walk you through them almost systematically. Some of the websites will help you compare the different types of abortions.

Some questions about abortion will be answered when you read the resources chapter and the associated websites and learn:

- How you can get help in paying for an abortion
- Where you can get an abortion in your area
- The surgical risks for each procedure and how those risks compare with the risks of a C-section or a vaginal delivery
- Whether your state requires you to notify the biological father or your parents before you have an abortion
- How long sperm lives so you can identify and notify the biological father, if necessary
- How to calculate how far along your pregnancy is
- How the fetus develops during the pregnancy
- Whether your state requires parental permission for a person your age to have an abortion
- Whether your state requires hospitalization for you to have certain types of abortions

Please remember that the field of medicine continues to advance, make discoveries, and perfect new techniques all the time. Some of what is written here might soon be out-of-date because of these changes. If you decide to have an abortion, your own doctor or the abortion provider are likely to be your best sources of the latest information. *Take what you read in this book as a starting point in your education.* One advantage of using chapter 7, "Abortion Resources," and going to the Internet sources is that some sites are revised continually.

# 5

## *Single Motherhood Resources*

There are many websites and books designed to interest single mothers. Some are commercially inspired, some are government sites, and others are nonprofit. Some sites are the work of single mothers and their supporters. I do not guarantee that any websites or books listed here are factual. These websites were last checked in 2015. Know that there may be more options for you than the ones offered on commercially backed websites. You will need to judge for yourself.

## Books and Book Lists

- *The Complete Single Mother: Reassuring Answers to Your Most Challenging Concerns* by Andrea Engber and Leah Klungness, PhD. The author has not read this book.

- *The Single Mother's Survival Guide* by Patrice Karst. The author has not read this book.

- Parentbooks is a Canadian website that lists books about single-parenting.
www.parentbooks.ca/Single_Parenting.html

- Find a short list of helpful books for single parenting on the Parents.com site:
  www.parents.com/fun/entertainment/books/single-parenting-books

- ASingleParents.com has a book list and other resources.
  www.asingleparents.com/books.html

## Some Costs of Single Motherhood

- You can get an idea of what your baby will cost you in the first year of his or her life by going to the BabyCenter website.
  www.babycenter.com/baby-cost-calculator

- You can get an estimate of what it cost to raise a child at these websites:
  www.babycenter.com/cost-of-raising-child-calculator
  www.cnpp.usda.gov/calculatorintro.htm

- As you consider single motherhood or adoption, you might want to weigh the risk of giving birth against the risks of having various kinds of abortions. To learn more about the risk of pregnancy and giving birth, go to the U.S. Centers for Disease Control and Prevention site. The CDC keeps track of deaths from complications of pregnancy. You can find their surveillance summary on pregnancy-related mortality from 1991–1999 online.
  www.cdc.gov/mmwr/preview/mmwrhtml/ss5202a1.htm

## Comprehensive Websites with Leads to Many Resources

- A group of single parents has put together helpful resources into one website. The website has useful articles, information, government resources, sitter locating, discussion forums, and book lists. They have an online group for parents to find friendships with other parents.
www.singleparentsnetwork.com

- Parents Without Partners is a nonprofit membership organization centered around helping single parents and their children by creating a supportive atmosphere where friendships and exchanges of techniques about parenting can occur.
www.parentswithoutpartners.org

- In an article called "50 Resources for Single Moms Going Back to College," the article's author has combed through many resources to find ones useful to single mothers seeking an education. Going back to school could make you feel better about you and improve your circumstances. This article lists websites and resources that can help you find legal information, a babysitter, money-saving coupons, single mother grants, travel opportunities, free items, discounts, financial help, and ways to share living arrangements. It lists several single mother blogs. This article includes a mechanism to match you to an online school. It lists sites where you can learn moneymaking crafts, gardening, cooking, housekeeping skills, and personal task management.
www.worldwidelearn.com/education-articles/
single-mom-resources.html

## Financial Assistance, Food Assistance, and Grants

Depending on where you live, you may get assistance through programs that help you pay your telephone bill, power bill, gas bill, water bill, and medical bills. You may get help with free weatherization and food. However, many people in need of these services may be competing with you. According to the United States Census Bureau, in 2011 there were ten million single mothers living with children younger than eighteen.

- The Need Help Paying Bills website offers some suggestions about how to utilize public, private, and commercial resources to pay various kinds of bills. It discusses help with taxes, mortgages, rent, credit card debt, and many more kinds of bills. It has a mechanism to learn about federal, state, and local government assistance programs.
  **www.needhelppayingbills.com**

- You may qualify for assistance from the federal government. The benefits website of the U.S. government can help you discover if you may be eligible for government benefits.
  **www.benefits.gov**

- Another site offers information about various government benefits, grants, and financial aid for U.S. citizens. This site links to many benefits, including weatherization assistance, renter's assistance, Temporary Assistance for Needy Families (TANF), food stamps, and health insurance for children.
  **www.usa.gov/Citizen/Topics/Benefits.shtml**

- The U.S. government has a program to offer nutritional assistance to low-income families called Supplemental Nutrition Assistance Program (SNAP).
www.fns.usda.gov/snap

- Find out whether you are eligible for the Special Supplemental Nutrition Program for Women, Infants, and Children (WIC). This program gives grants to states so they can provide "supplemental foods, health-care referrals, nutrition education for low-income pregnant, breastfeeding, nonbreast-feeding postpartum women, and to infants and children up to age five found at nutritional risk."
www.fns.usda.gov/wic/women-infants-and-children-wic

- One Harvest is an organization that distributes affordable prepackaged, preordered food in boxes through their partner sites once a month. You may call them at 770-466-0000 or go to their website.
www.oneharvest.com

- You can find a food bank close to you at the Feeding America website:
www.feedingamerica.org/find-your-local-foodbank

## Money Management

- Consider going to a credit counselor. Remember that some credit counselors that label themselves as nonprofit are not. Get help with picking a credit counselor.
www.consumer.ftc.gov/articles/
  0153-choosing-credit-counselor

If possible, encourage the biological father to buy life insurance on his life that would pay his child in case of his early death. This insurance would help replace his child support in the event of his death. You should buy life insurance as well if you can.

- You need health insurance. You can find out about the Affordable Healthcare Act and about Medicaid eligibility by consulting two websites.
  www.hhs.gov/healthcare
  www.medicaid.gov

## Saving Money

- CoAbode is a website that matches single moms with one or more children with other single moms so they can share housing, resources, and finances. Through the help of donations, CoAbode is free to all single mothers. This site has other resources as well.
  www.coabode.org

- You may find inexpensive clothes, furniture, books, and other items at Goodwill. Goodwill also offers help with finding jobs. For immediate help in finding a job call 800-GOODWILL or go to their website.
  www.goodwill.org/find-jobs-and-services

## Sharing

Buy food in bulk with someone else and split the cost. Use a food cooperative. Ask your friends to think of you when they have an extra ticket to an activity. If you do not have a computer, use your public library. Pay bills online to avoid the cost of stamps. Eat with friends and volunteer to take the leftovers. If you have friends with children a little older than your own child is, offer to buy their hand-me-down clothes. Carpool to save gas and maintenance on your car. Share housing.

## Bartering

Instead of buying something with money, try bartering. Exchange your services (like cleaning, cooking, babysitting) for something you want. Move in with an elderly person (your elderly aunt?) who needs help or companionship in exchange for not having to pay rent. You could also barter for the service of another person (like a college co-ed) who would stay with you and take care of your child by letting her stay with you rent-free.

## Avoiding Paying Full Price

Use coupons. Wait for sales. Buy on layaway. Buy off-season. Buy in bulk. Buy store brands. Buy generic drugs. Buy at yard or garage sales. If an item is damaged or dirty, ask the store manager for a discount. Postpone buying until you can pay with cash to avoid interest charges. Ask if there is a discount for paying cash (stores have to pay a fee if you use a credit card). Pay your credit cards down to avoid paying interest.

## Avoiding Extra Expenses

Move closer to where you work to save gas and time. If you move into a city, you might access several services more easily and, by taking the subway or bus or train, you can avoid paying for a car.

Avoid paying extra expenses for nonessentials like cigarettes and alcohol. Pets can be wonderful but expensive. Pets require food, medical care, added deposits for rentals, and your time. Avoid costly accidents by childproofing your house and resolving to drive safely. Make sure everyone in your car always uses a seat belt or car seat.

If you have poor credit, you will pay higher interest rates. You can establish credit by paying off your credit card monthly. You will have a better chance of being able to do this if you avoid buying unnecessary items. If you have bad credit, look at the website in this chapter about credit counseling.

Avoid unnecessary medical expenses by taking good care of your health. Wash your hands before you touch your lips, eyes, or mouth to avoid getting sick and missing work. Make sure you are not anemic or have some untreated illness that makes you feel tired and less productive. Preventing illness, or treating it early, is eventually cheaper.

Reduce the risk of getting pregnant with a second child by using effective contraception. See the resources at the end of chapter 7, "Abortion Resources."

## Doing It Yourself

Try raising your own food in a backyard garden. Use some sites mentioned in this chapter to learn to cook so you can spend less on fast food. Some sites in this chapter link to programs where women teach other women auto repair skills.

## Thinking Creatively About Making Money

Make sure you get the child support due you from the biological father. Do DNA testing. Go back to court if you have to. For a small extra fee, some Departments of Family and Children Services will let him pay them and they pay you. This keeps track of his payments. It is to your advantage to encourage the biological father to get more education so he is in a better position to pay you child support.

Resell good, used clothing in consignment or thrift stores. Have yard sales.

Think of how some of your skills may help you make money. Tutor students. Give art lessons. Give music lessons. Cook. Use your craft skills to make items you can sell on consignment. Assemble things. Paint paintings. Paint houses. Knit. Bake wedding cakes. Teach softball. Look for odd jobs on Craigslist. Help students with papers. Be the neighborhood babysitter for several children.

Look at the sites that talk about working from home, but be careful to avoid the scams. Consider the more established companies that let you sell things.

Remember, working seasonal employment may help you. When your employer is hiring permanent employees, your boss already knows the quality of your work.

## Taking Care of You

Taking care of yourself requires planning. It involves sharing duties, finding ways to take breaks, creating affordable entertainment, setting limits on others to minimize unnecessary work, and paying attention to your emotional needs. Here are a hodgepodge of ideas to start you brainstorming about this.

By networking with other single mothers, you can learn of opportunities to relieve them by sitting for their children, and they can do the same for you another time.

Lose excessive weight to reduce the energy it takes for you to do daily activities. Learn about healthy eating:
**www.nutrition.gov**

Do things that may be entertaining but are also free. Go to high school plays. Go to church programs. Watch your local school's ball teams. Go to public concerts in the park. Just play with your child and enjoy the bonding experience.

Think about how you can work smarter, not harder, by doing things more effectively. Making your child feel more secure by having a daily routine will also give you a sense of steadiness. Make a plan for the day.

Taking care of you and preserving energy sometimes requires setting limits on people who take advantage of your wish to please them. Consider using the Iron Rule more often: "Do not do for others what they can do for themselves." Refuse other adults who make excessive demands for your efforts or time.

Delegate responsibility then follow up. Accept that others may not do it the way you like, but you do not have to do it. You no longer have the time to do everything yourself and be in control. Figure out who you can count on, and try to count on them.

Join a single mother support group. Find a mentor.

If your parents are helping you, consider moving closer to where they live. If your mother has a day job, consider working evenings so she can watch your child. The closer your home, your sitter's home, and your place of work are, the less time you spend on the road. Think about ways to shorten your day.

Besides addressing ways to take care of yourself as you cope with everyday stressors, you need to think about the emotional stressors. These are less visible and may be harder to identify when you are so busy.

Part of taking care of you is reaching out for help when you recognize that you feel depressed, anxious, and overwhelmed. Most counties have community mental health clinics that operate on a sliding scale or take Medicaid. In addition, there are churches and other community organizations that can offer counseling.

- After you deliver, if you think your baby blues are too intense or lasting too long, you may want to read this article on postpartum depression: www.nlm.nih.gov/medlineplus/ency/article/007215.htm

- If you feel suicidal, it is very important that you get help immediately. Don't wait. Call the National Suicide Hotline any time at 1-800-273-8255.

- You may find it helpful to read *Choosing to Live: How to Defeat Suicide Through Cognitive Therapy* by Dr. Thomas Ellis and Dr. Cory Newman.

## Preparing to Date Again

If you want to date again, you can find information about dating by looking at the websites and books mentioned in this chapter. Deciding whether to date again is a complex personal decision. Your life might be easier with the right partner, and worse with the wrong one.

If you feel reluctant to start dating, you might try going to Parents Without Partners group activities with your child.

Please realize that, if you are an attractive woman, some men are too intimidated by you to approach you. If your warm smile doesn't do it, approach them.

As mentioned earlier, it is not simply having a man around but having the right man around that benefits your child. Better to have no man around than to have the wrong man.

One example of the wrong man would be a sexual predator. If a boyfriend is not that interested in you sexually, think again.

- You can get help in determining the sexual predators living near you or search for them by name on the U.S. Department of Justice's website:
  www.nsopr.gov

## Helping Your Child Get More Fathering

Enlist your male friends. Get your dad involved. As your child grows, put him or her around trusted schoolteachers, teachers at your place of worship, school bandleaders, ball coaches, or neighbors.

- Peer Resources has a website that lists various kinds of mentoring programs in the United States, Canada, and the United Kingdom.
  www.peer.ca/mentorprograms.html

You may want to take the time to search the Internet for a local mentoring program for you or your child. Local organizations and schools set up many mentoring programs.

- When your child turns six, consider joining Big Brothers Big Sisters, which provides one-to-one mentoring for children age 6–18.
  www.bbbs.org

When your child is older, consider Boys & Girls Clubs, Boy Scouts of America, Girl Scouts of the USA, the YMCA, and the YWCA.

## Being Approachable

Your attitude has a big effect on whether people are willing to help you. Work at overcoming shyness and pride so you can reach out for help when you need it. Your child cannot afford for you to be shy or fall into bitter victimhood. People are more willing to help if they know you. How can they know you if you do not show up and participate in the group? Sometimes groups will have a nursery for members so parents can attend more easily.

When people do something for you, try to give back. Show gratitude. Send them a thank-you note. Bake them some cookies. Take your turn at working in the group's nursery.

- Check out "How to Be More Approachable":
  www.wikihow.com/Be-More-Approachable

## Getting More Education and Job Skills

Google "typing" to access free typing instruction. Search online at Google.com or another search engine for "resume preparation" to access sites offering help with writing a résumé. Consider applying for the Pell Grant, federal aid for low-income college students. Look for other scholarships for single mothers. Take online courses from home.

Be careful about for-profit (sometimes called "proprietary") colleges. While some of these colleges are very good and will prepare you to earn a living, others are not. A regional accrediting group should accredit the entire college.

- See an explanation of accreditation:
  www.en.wikipedia.org/wiki/Regional_accreditation

Sometimes specific programs are accredited by other organizations, but if the college or university isn't accredited overall, your degree might not allow you to go into the field that you want. Look into the percentage of graduates who get jobs in the career that you want to enter.

In addition to getting more career education, it is important for you to educate yourself about parenting and child development. Read about parenting. Talk to other mothers. Study parenting skills so it is easier for you to be a good parent. You will have fewer problems later if you make fewer child-rearing mistakes now. Work on age-appropriate child responsibility. Set limits. Children will try to rise to your expectations. As your child grows older, you should expect more of him or her, within reason.

# 6

## Adoption Resources

You will see from going to the websites in this chapter that adoptive parents must be quite motivated to adopt a child. Potential adoptive parents must go through a home study inspection, submit to a criminal records search, take parenting classes, undergo interviews with agency staff, interview with you as the birth mother if you want, and wait a number of months. Some adoptive parents may spend thousands of dollars in fees.

Adoptive parents are asked to submit histories about their past marriages and why they ended in divorce, religious preferences and religious involvement, children from previous marriages, occupations, annual income, health problems, career plans, racial makeup, sexual preferences, whether they will take time off after the adoption, and the desired level of openness they want with the biological parents.

### An Overview

American Adoptions is an adoption agency whose website can be used to provide an overview of adoption. This website explains the adoption process in detail. It discusses how financial help varies with the state you are in, your living situation, and how far along you are in your pregnancy.

It covers how to discuss adoption with the birth father, how adoptive families are screened, and the advantages of adoption. It answers frequently asked questions, discusses adoption requirements for birth mothers, and explains legal services. It lists free services for pregnant mothers like adoption counseling. The website discusses the differences between open, closed, and semi-open adoptions. It discusses how to deal with various kinds of situations with the birth father and with the birth mother's potentially unsupportive parents.

The website discusses the advantages of telling supportive people about your situation but explains how you could move to another town if you have pressing needs to keep your pregnancy or adoption secret. It discusses how you might approach telling your parents.

It quotes some statistics to examine the health and happiness of adopted children and the benefits of open adoptions. American Adoptions says that they offer scholarships each year to selected women who want to further their education.

- You can ask American Adoptions staff your questions about adoption by filling out a form on their website or calling them. Call 1-800-ADOPTION or go to their website:
  www.americanadoptions.com

Most states have a Division of Family and Children Services (DFACS), usually listed under the Department of Human Resources. It may offer you information about adoption in your state.

Several studies have been conducted on the effect the openness of the adoption has on the well-being of the adopted child and the adoptive family. Three of these studies are noted later in this chapter. A detailed reading of them is well worth your time.

## Adoption Agencies

In addition to American Adoptions, many other adoption agencies have websites that do a good job of answering practical questions about adoption. The adoption agency or independent adoption service that you pick may depend on where you live. Each state has different laws about adoption. Adoption agencies are limited in what they can provide based on these laws. Some sites that address some of your basic questions about adoption are listed in this chapter.

- To find an adoption agency in your state, use Google or another Internet search engine to search for "licensed adoption agencies in [your state]."

- You can find the names and ratings of adoption agencies online:
  www.adoptionagencyratings.com

## Independent Adoptions

- The Independent Adoption Center is an open adoption agency. IAC is a nonprofit organization that provides support for adoptive parents and women considering adoption.
  www.adoptionhelp.org

The website discusses the Minnesota/Texas Adoption Research Project, the California Long-Range Adoption Study, and the Open Adoption of Infants research by D. H. Siegel.

    The Independent Adoption Center also lists adoption

websites and covers general information, adoption law, and adoption forums.

- An open adoption agency that focuses on connecting adoptive parents and children of color is Pact. The Pact website has several general articles about adoption as well. www.pactadopt.org

## Adoption Law

- Legal Match, a website that refers attorneys, has an article online that discusses the rights the birth father has in the adoption:
www.legalmatch.com/law-library/article/
  adoption-and-fathers-rights.html

- The U.S. Department of Health & Human Services operates the Child Welfare Information Gateway. This website allows you to search the adoption laws in your state to answer questions about fathers' rights, access to adoption records, adoption expenses, adoption procedures, and other topics.
www.childwelfare.gov/topics/systemwide/laws-policies/state

## Maternity Homes

A maternity home is a living environment that may also provide a variety of supportive services to pregnant women who, for whatever the reason, are unable to have a stable place to stay for the rest of their pregnancy.

- ABC Adoptions maintains a small nationwide list of maternity homes on their website.
www.abcadoptions.com/maternityhomes.htm

- The website Adoption.com discusses birth mother housing.
  www.adoption.com/housing

- To find a list of programs awarded grants for transitional living and maternity group homes go to the Family & Youth Services Bureau website (maintained by the U.S. Department of Health & Human Services). In the site's search box type "2014 Transitional Living and Maternity Group Home Awards." This will not bring up the document in detail, but you will be able to see the list of the maternity homes near you that were given grants.
  www.acf.hhs.gov/programs/fysb

## Choosing an Adoptive Family

You can get information about the state requirements for people to become adoptive parents by searching at Google for "Frequently Asked Questions about adoption in Alabama." The search results will give you answers for the state of Alabama. Substitute the name of your state for the word "Alabama." Then scroll down the list of results to the website you want to visit.
  www.google.com

- Choosing an adoptive family for your child is a most important decision that affects you, your child, and the adoptive family. Adoption agencies can be one source of support as you evaluate prospective adoptive parents. Consider the possibility of sharing your selection-making process with those who love you. The Family Formation, an adoption agency, offers a discussion about choosing an adoptive family:
  www.familyformation.com/choosing-an-adoptive-family

## Adoption Scams

- My Adoption Advisor, an agency for adoptive parents, discusses adoption scams and how to avoid them:
  www.myadoptionadvisor.com/th-gallery/adoption-scams-fraud/

## Teen Pregnancy

- The American College of Obstetricians and Gynecology answers frequently asked questions about teen pregnancy.
  www.acog.org/Patients/FAQs/Pregnancy-Having-a-Baby-Especially-for-Teens

## Contraception

Information about contraception is contained in the next chapter, "Abortion Resources."

# 7

## *Abortion Resources*

Use these many resources to educate yourself about abortion.

### Seeking Answers About Your Pregnancy

- Backline has a pregnancy talkline at 1-888-493-0092. Their website states, "Backline promotes unconditional and judgment-free support for people in all their decisions, feelings, and experiences with pregnancy, adoption, and abortion."
www.yourbackline.org

- You can look at the size and length of the developing fetus at TheBump.com. This site notes that the fetus is, on average, .63 inches long at 8 weeks, 2.1 inches long at 12 weeks, 4.6 inches long at 16 weeks, 6.5 inches long at 20 weeks, and 10.5 inches long at 24 weeks gestation.
http://pregnant.thebump.com/pregnancy-week-by-week.aspx

- The American College of Obstetricians and Gynecologists answers frequently asked questions about pregnancy options.
www.acog.org/Patients/FAQs/Pregnancy-Choices-Raising-the-Baby-Adoption-and-Abortion

- The Before Abortion website sells *The Before Abortion Audio Workbook*, a "pro-choice counseling session for women who want to work through their thoughts and feelings before making a choice about a pregnancy." This site also has free self-tests and offers links to other resources.
  www.beforeandafterabortion.com

## Determining How Far Along You Are

- The information in the article "Sperm: How long do they live after ejaculation?" may help you understand the factors involved in determining the biological father if you have had several partners.
  www.mayoclinic.org/pregnancy/expert-answers/faq-20058504

- In determining how long you have been pregnant (called the *gestational age*), you may want to use the interactive Pregnancy Information Tool provided by Premier Diagnostic Services, Inc. Just click on the wheel to move the tool.
  www.premierus.com/dynamic-pregnancy-wheel

- A pregnancy conception calculator attempts to determine your date of conception based on your last menstrual period, ovulation, or ultrasound. Go to BabyMed and enter your estimate of your usual menstrual cycle length and last menstrual period. Based on your *estimated* date of conception, you can determine who is most likely to be the biological father.
  www.babymed.com/conception-calculator

If you have an abortion, your abortion provider will do an ultrasound to determine the gestational age of the fetus before a procedure will be done. (An ultrasound machine safely bounces sound waves off the fetus to make a computer-generated picture of the fetus.) This is important because the gestational age will determine what kind of procedure can be done, and *women sometimes are mistaken about the gestational age.*

The article "Accuracy of Gestational Age Estimated by Menstrual Dating in Women Seeking Abortion Beyond Nine Weeks" appeared in the *Journal of Obstetrics Gynaecology of Canada*. The article concluded, "Women seeking surgical abortion for pregnancies of 9–20 weeks underreport gestational age by an average of 1.2 weeks using menstrual dating." They found that the farther along the woman was, the more discrepancy there was between the estimated gestational age and the age determined from using an ultrasound machine.

## Medical Abortion

This book provides only a brief overview of abortion procedures and related medical issues. This book is not intended to take the place of your having a serious discussion with your health care provider. **If you are considering an abortion, talk with a licensed health care provider right away.** Make the effort to visit the websites listed in this chapter and other chapters to build the kind of in-depth understanding that you need to make your best decision.

- Medline Plus, a program of the U.S. National Institutes of Health, provides a wide range of health information. You can find their article on medical abortion here: www.nlm.nih.gov/medlineplus/ency/article/007382.htm

- An article on WebMD discusses mifepristone and misoprostol for abortion
  www.webmd.com/women/
    mifepristone-and-misoprostol-for-abortion

## Surgical Abortion

- You can find a detailed, systematic description of the manual and vacuum aspiration methods of abortion on WebMD. (A free, onetime registration is required in order to review the entire article and all other content on the Medscape and WebMD websites.)
  www.webmd.com/women/
    manual-and-vacuum-aspiration-for-abortion

- The National Abortion Federation has a table that compares advantages and disadvantages of the different types of first trimester abortions. (This site also has a discussion of mifepristone.) Download the table here:
  www.prochoice.org/wp-content/uploads/comparison_first_
    trimester.pdf

- MedlinePlus has articles about surgical abortion and after-care following a surgical abortion.
  www.nlm.nih.gov/medlineplus/ency/article/002912.htm
  www.nlm.nih.gov/medlineplus/ency/
    patientinstructions/000658.htm

- Medscape also has useful articles on general gynecology topics, general obstetrical topics, abortion, labor and delivery, and others.
  http://emedicine.medscape.com/obstetrics_gynecology

## Examples of Specific Provider Websites

You will find useful information on any number of abortion provider websites. I list these two as examples, not intending to make any promises about the websites' or providers' usefulness, accuracy, or timeliness.

On their website, Planned Parenthood of Southeastern Virginia writes that vacuum aspiration surgical abortions are performed in most cases up to sixteen weeks after a woman's last period, and dilatation and evacuation surgical abortions are performed after that. They note that, after twenty-four weeks of pregnancy, abortions are not done except for "serious health reasons."

- This website explains how each type of abortion is done, discusses the surgical risks, talks about what you could expect right after the abortion, and makes some estimates of the cost of a first trimester abortion.
  www.ppsev.org/our-services/pregnancy-options/abortion-options/

Northland Family Planning has clinics located around the Detroit metropolitan area. On their website they report that they do two kinds of vacuum aspiration. They discuss at what gestational ages they do manual vacuum aspiration, standard vacuum aspiration, and the dilation and evacuation procedure.

- The Northland Family Planning website has an "After abortion video" to educate you about what to look for after your abortion. The Northland Family Planning website offers a link to another video, "Everyday Good Women," and they have a blog as well.
  www.northlandfamilyplanning.com

- A free workbook that can help you with decision making is *Pregnancy Options Workbook* by Margaret Johnston.
  www.pregnancyoptions.info/pregnantPrint.htm

## Finding a Provider

The author has not personally reviewed or investigated the providers you may find through these sites, and you should carefully research any provider you consider using.

- You can use Planned Parenthood's Health Center Searcher to find an abortion provider.
  www.plannedparenthood.org/health-center

- The National Abortion Federation (NAF) offers a national provider search. This search function also will tell you about any special conditions that might be required in your particular state to get an abortion. Some states require a waiting period after you have seen an abortion provider. Some states require you to notify a parent (if you are younger than 18) or receive counseling with state-specified materials. The site also has a hotline for help in finding a provider, and a separate phone number to learn about financial assistance available in some cases.
  www.prochoice.org/think-youre-pregnant/find-a-provider

- The Abortion Care Network (ACN), a nonprofit organization of independent abortion providers and allies, will also help you locate a provider. Call them at 1-202-419-1444 or e-mail them at info@abortioncarenetwork.org as well as visiting their website.
  www.abortioncarenetwork.org/clinics

## Paying for the Abortion

The cost of an abortion varies. It depends on several things such as the kind of procedure done, your insurance coverage, and the state in which you live.

- The National Abortion Federation publishes a fact sheet that discusses abortion costs.
  www.prochoice.org/education-and-advocacy/about-abortion/abortion-facts/#dea44672e76df75e3

- For information and financial assistance with an abortion, call the National Abortion Federation hotline at 1-800-772-9100.

- The National Network of Abortion Funds also offers help in finding funding. They also have a list of the states that cover abortion services for low-income women under Medicaid if the abortion is termed necessary medically.
  www.fundabortionnow.org

The National Network of Abortion Funds website also gives suggestions on how to produce some money on your own to put with the money you might get from an abortion fund.

Some abortion clinics and providers will allow discounts, accept credit cards, or work out payment plans. Planned Parenthood will accept several kinds of insurance and may also treat women who do not have insurance.

## The Fetal Pain Issue

- You may have found a variety of websites that talk about whether the fetus experiences pain during an abortion. An article by Joyce Arthur, "Fetal Pain: A Red Herring in the Abortion Debate," addresses this issue.
  www.prochoiceactionnetwork-canada.org/articles/fetal-pain.shtml

## The Emotional Effects Issue

Single motherhood, adoption, and abortion can all cause emotional distress. Opinions differ widely about how much emotional distress abortion causes. If you're not sure how distressful it would be for you to have an abortion, you might find it helpful to read various opinions, starting with the resources in this section. Some resources suggest that the amount of emotional distress is best predicted by how well you were doing mentally before the abortion. Other resources suggest that it would not be unusual even for mentally healthy women to have some common emotional responses.

- The National Abortion Federation, in copyrighted material from their website, discusses on their website the scientific research on how having an abortion affects the woman having it. The NAF notes, "Mainstream medical opinions, like that of the American Psychological Association, agree there is no such thing as a 'post-abortion syndrome.'"
  www.prochoice.org/education-and-advocacy/about-abortion/abortion-myths

The NAF cites an eight-year study as concluding that "the most important predictor of emotional well-being in post-abortion women was their well-being before the abortion."

*Because your well-being is such a strong predictor, have you discussed your current emotional state with those closest to you? Please don't skip this step in your decision process.*

The NAF points out that while having an abortion can be stressful, there is stress involved in adoption and unwanted childbearing as well.

- Dr. Nada Logan Stotland, MD, former president of the American Psychiatric Association, wrote an article for *The Huffington Post* called "Abortion Trauma: The Myth." A consideration of your situation is incomplete without reading this thoughtful article.
www.huffingtonpost.com/nada-logan-stotland-md-mph/abortion-trauma-syndrome-b_776342.html

## Emotional Support After the Abortion

Even though research suggests that women who are mentally healthy before the abortion usually don't have long-term psychological problems from having the procedure, they can experience a range of emotions right after the abortion that can be helped by emotional support. Here are some resources.

- ImNotSorry.net is a site "where women can share stories about their positive experiences with abortion."
www.imnotsorry.net

- Exhale offers a free, national talkline (1-866-4-EXHALE) providing post-abortion counseling in multiple languages. They also support friends, family, and loved ones of the person who had an abortion.
  www.exhaleprovoice.org

- There is a support group "for those who have terminated a pregnancy for nonmedical reasons and for women highly considering terminating for nonmedical reasons" at BabyCenter.com.
  http://community.babycenter.com/groups/a7815/termination_for_non-medical_reasons

- The National Abortion Federation also discusses how to take care of yourself after the abortion and also offers book suggestions and other resources.
  www.prochoice.org/think-youre-pregnant/what-should-i-expect-after-the-abortion

## The Laws in Your State About Abortion

The Guttmacher Institute website, Gutmacher.org, provides an overview of abortion laws and each state's abortion policy in brief, including the requirements and restrictions that it places on abortion. Your state may require counseling, a waiting period, or parental involvement. Some states restrict how abortions can be funded. Other states limit who can perform abortions, where they can be performed, and when they can be performed. You should independently check the law in your state.

There are some restrictions on when abortion can be performed. This varies from state to state and depends on how the particular state defines "viability, or when the fetus could reasonably be expected to survive on its own outside the mother's uterus." For example, some states legally define it as twenty weeks, and others as twenty-four weeks.

- The Guttmacher Institute's overview of abortion laws is available here:
  www.guttmacher.org/statecenter/spibs/spib_OAL.pdf

## Contraception

- A medication or device that prevents pregnancy is called a contraceptive. You can reduce the risk of getting pregnant with another child by using effective contraception. The WomensHealth.gov website provides information about the various types of contraception.
  www.womenshealth.gov/publications/our-publications/
    fact-sheet/birth-control-methods.html

- Planned Parenthood also provides a discussion of various types of birth control.
  www.plannedparenthood.org/health-info/birth-control

- The Guttmacher Institute provide a fact sheet about contraception and contraceptive effectiveness on their website.
  www.guttmacher.org/pubs/fb_contr_use.html

- The Eunice Kennedy Shriver National Institute of Child Health and Human Development website offers another discussion of the various types of contraceptives. www.nichd.nih.gov/health/topics/contraception/conditioninfo/pages/types.aspx

# 8

## *Conclusion*

There are women all over the world experiencing unplanned pregnancies right now. Because you may not know any of them, you may feel alone. If you do know other women with unplanned pregnancies, reach out to them!

You can see from the resource chapters of this book that many people care about you and about what you are experiencing. They are ready to help you. Reach out to them!

Have you made this book the beginning of a continuing discussion with the people who accept and love you? Reach out to them!

Do you believe God is like a steadfast, loving parent who is with you in your distress and wants the best for you? Reach out to God!

Have courage. You are not alone. Reach out!

# Appendix

# A-1

## *The Biological Father*

Even though the biological father is more complex than any stereotype, it is difficult to talk about the typical behavior of men and women without stereotypes.

If your pregnancy makes you feel as though you also have to decide about your relationship with the biological father, these books may help:

- *The Hard Questions: 100 Questions to Ask Before You Say "I Do"* by Susan Piver

- *Too Good to Leave, Too Bad to Stay: A Step-by-Step Guide to Help You Decide Whether to Stay In or Get Out of Your Relationship* by Mira Kirshenbaum

The ideal partner will be passionate, permanent, partner-ready, problem-solving, parent-material, productive, personable, and protective. Yet partners are just human. It's okay if the biological father doesn't pass all the questions in this chapter. The essential question for you: Does the biological father pass enough of them for you to bring a child into the relationship?

## Passionate

Do you love the biological father? Does he love you? Are you a priority in his life? Is your child a priority as well? Some men step up to fatherhood while others just aren't ready. Can you make a clear decision about his passion to be a dad?

## Permanent

Can you count on your relationship to be permanent? Has he a dangerous occupation that could result in his death? Is he in good health? Does he have a history of being unfaithful in past relationships?

If you cannot count on the biological father, do you have a father, grandfather, other close male relative, or best male friend who could provide some fathering for your child? If you died suddenly, is there someone else who could raise your child if the biological father could not?

## Partner-Ready

Is the biological father ready to be an active partner in raising your child? What examples of him making sacrifices for others might make you think he would make sacrifices for your child?

How he treats others, especially people like his mother and those in a service role (like store clerks, secretaries, or waiters), may give you a clue about how he will treat you and your child. Have you seen him be kind, considerate, helpful, and loving to his mother in various situations over a long period?

A good partner accepts advice from his mate. Can you think of examples where he has accepted advice from his dad or from his boss? Can he accept advice from women as well as men?

Does he look at life the same way you do? Do you believe

the same things? Do you think you would be able to agree on how to parent? Do you have the same dreams?

## Problem-Solving

Is the biological father a problem solver? Has he shown intelligence, persistence, and the ability to tolerate frustration when he tries to solve problems? How have you worked together to solve problems?

## Parent-Material

Will he be able to be close to your child?

Will he put you and your child first? Has he other obligations that make you and your child a lower priority?

How has he done at child-care experiences like babysitting, working at camp, or taking care of brothers and sisters? Is he a responsible pet owner? How does he respond in situations around other people's loud, needy, messy children?

## Productive

Has he the skills and personality that he needs to keep a job and be a productive provider for you and your child? If he has difficulty in taking responsibility for his mistakes and always blames his boss, he may have problems keeping a job. Does he have a legal history that will hold him back?

## Personable

When you are in love, it is easy to overlook things in your partner or think you can change his personality with your love and care. After all his years of being a certain way, it may be quite difficult for your partner to change his views and approach to daily life.

Is he ordinarily happy and satisfied with life or is he always down on himself? If he views himself as a victim, will he start to blame you and your child for holding him back?

Does the biological father think about others or is he self-centered? If he is demanding, will he become jealous when you show attention to your "other child"?

What evidence do you have that the biological father has the ability to trust? If the biological father is suspicious of you despite your efforts to earn his trust, he might also have trouble having a close, trusting relationship with your child.

Is the biological father honest and trustworthy? For example, does he tell you what you want to hear to avoid conflict? If you have talked about your pregnancy, did he say what you wanted to hear although he actually wants something different instead?

Does the biological father exercise self-control by saying no to himself or his friends when necessary? Would he make impulsive decisions that would affect you and your child?

## Protective

Is the biological father looking out for you? Has he been protective of you, or do you feel worried about being protected from him? Has he been violent toward you? Has he isolated you from your friends, shown unjustified jealousy, or bullied you? Would he bully your child? Will living with the biological father place your child around unpredictable people who make your child feel insecure? Would you be living in an unsafe neighborhood? Would you have to live with a partner or his relatives who are unstable because of their addictions or mental illness?

Do you feel safe telling the biological father that you are

pregnant? Would the biological father feel uncontrollably angry, trapped, or desperate if he knew that you were pregnant and were thinking about keeping the baby?

*Go back now and ask these questions about you.* Do any of the descriptions fit you? How would that affect your ability to be a single mother?

Besides the qualities you are examining about the biological father, there may be complicated situations that you need to address related to the biological father and your relationship.

## Secrets

Are you worried that having an abortion, having a baby, or proceeding with an adoption would negatively affect your relationship? Do you want to consider first what you want to do before you ask his opinion?

If you have an abortion and never tell the biological father, how will such a secret affect your relationship? If you remain pregnant and go past the time that you could have had an abortion before telling him, is it fair to commit him to paying child support for eighteen or more years without his knowledge or permission?

## Unhappily Married

Perhaps you are already married and have been thinking about leaving your husband. In that situation, will having a child make it impossible to leave? Will deciding to have your child result in your being trapped in an abusive relationship?

## His Parents

Will his parents help? Do they like you? Will they mind your taking resources from their son and from them? Will they be upset if they see you interfering with their son's completing school, getting ahead in his job, and so on? Are you going to be fighting your child's grandparents for years over custody of your child?

## Inherited Diseases

Will your child be at risk of inheriting a mental illness from the biological father that may make your child more difficult to live with or to raise, such as a mood disorder or thinking disorder? Is the biological father capable of raising a special-needs child?

If the adoption agency knew about a hereditary defect or mental illness in the biological father's family, would that make it difficult for them to place your child with an adoptive family?

## Your Husband Is Not the Biological Father

If you have become pregnant by someone other than your husband, would your husband's knowing that end your marriage? Would your husband be able to raise another man's child? Unusual situations like your child needing a kidney or a blood transfusion could reveal that your child is not your husband's child.

# A-2

## Supplementary Questions About Single Motherhood

The additional information and more detailed questions in this chapter may help clarify your thinking about single motherhood.

You may be determined that, if you ever decide to be a mother, you will work to be a better mother to your child than your mother was to you. For one reason or another, being mothered by your mother may not have been a positive loving experience for you. When someone talks about the mother-child relationship, your first response may be sadness.

### The Joys of Single Motherhood

If you have been fortunate enough to have a positive relationship with your mother, you may have always thought you would be a mother. Do you look forward to teaching your child about the world and life? Do you get excited when you think about the warmth and closeness you will have with your child? Do you like the idea of feeling needed and respected by your child? Are you thinking you can count on your child to love you and stay with you in a way you cannot depend on with men? Do you feel having a child will give you purpose and direction in your life? Do you look forward to watching your child grow up?

If you have had a good relationship with your mom and have had a happy childhood, the joys of single motherhood may be obvious to you. Perhaps the question for you is not whether you want a baby. You may be sure that you do. Your real question may be "Is it best to have the baby now and with this partner?"

## Positive Alternatives to Having a Child

Our culture naturally reinforces parenthood to continue civilization. However, without women who decide not to have children, our civilization would lose some of its richness.

Some pursuits may require a single-minded devotion that makes good parenting very difficult. The sciences, arts, music, drama, medicine, literature, journalism, research, and many other fields all benefit from the dedication of women who have decided to give their lives to helping society in other ways. Mothers and their children benefit every day in subtle ways from women who have decided not to have children themselves.

Could *you* be the aunt who is such a presence in the lives of your nieces and nephews, and such a help to your sister or brother? Could you be the teacher or coach to whom teenagers will listen when they cannot hear a thing their parents say?

Could you be the pediatric nurse who watches over a child at night while the worried mother sleeps? Could you be the mother to your handicapped parent who frees your sister up to take care of your nieces and nephews? These are some of many ways for you to express your love for children.

## Single Mothering Skills

What skills have you developed from looking after other people's children or your brothers and sisters? Were you good at teaching children when you tutored? Did you find you had a way with children as a camp counselor? Did your mother teach you homemaking skills, so that you already know how to budget, cook, and clean? Did your mom and dad provide good models for parenting?

Were you the one at family gatherings who always had the baby in your lap or were playing with the children outside? Do your niece and nephew beg to spend overnights with you?

Can you amuse the fussy child in the doctor's office or standing in line in front of you? Does the family look to you to calm your brother or sister? Do people kid you that you treat your dog as though it were your child and take better care of it than they would?

Are you good at putting off getting something you want then accepting a less expensive brand when you do get it? Do friends praise you for your ability to stick with difficult things until you finish them?

Are you good at cooperating with others and getting them to work with you on tasks? Are you good about asking for help when you need it? Do people tell you that you are realistic in what you think you can do?

Having self-doubts is usual when you are preparing to do something for the first time. Do you think you could take some time to learn some things during your pregnancy that would help you feel more prepared to be a single mother?

## The Effect of Your Single Motherhood on Others

If you think your parents will need to help you, then how well do you and your parents work with each other?

Will you be able to spend enough time with your infant in the beginning to form the crucial early bonding? If not, will your baby end up bonding to your mother as his or her mother?

Children experience emotional deprivation when conditions do not permit enough or adequate interpersonal interaction. Will you be able to provide enough interpersonal interaction between the time you provide and the time others provide? That is, will the child be in a situation that allows them to form a close, secure relationship with you and develop trust in your ability to care for them?

You are taking a risk when you don't make sure you know what your parents (or partner) think and feel as soon as possible. After all, if you were to put off talking with them about your decisions until you were too far along in your pregnancy to get an abortion and you didn't want to put your child up for adoption, you would be making decisions without their knowledge that might seriously affect their life.

On the other hand, if you underestimate their willingness to help you raise your child or go through the adoption process, you may have an abortion that you might have rejected if you had only known.

Do you know what your family's financial situation is? Maybe they are doing well and could help you without much impact on them. Maybe they have secure jobs and are not worried about losing them.

On the other hand, is it possible that their helping you would result in their having a lower standard of living, being unable to help your siblings or grandparents, having to work more hours, having to put off their retirement, having to go into debt, or having to help you when they had other plans for their time?

How old will your parents be when your child is ten, seventeen, and twenty-one? What is your guess about what their health will be like then?

Six years from now, will family members who want to help still have the physical and mental ability to think clearly, show good judgment, and be responsible when they are left alone with your child? Will they still have what it takes to handle a teenager thirteen years from now?

## Handling Stress

Are you good at accepting that you have done something the best you can and at not feeling guilty when you don't have the time or energy you think you should for your child? Are you able to avoid dwelling on the fact that you're missing what others your age are doing? Can you instead focus on discovering the world through your child's eyes? Are you naturally unselfish and giving? Do your friends comment on how mature and grown-up you are?

If being poor means that your child does not have the basic opportunities that other children have, then being poor has affected your child. Will you be able to make up to your child with your love and attention for the opportunities he or she may not have?

Just because single motherhood may be hard on *you* does not necessarily mean you should not do it, so long as it being hard on you has minimal impact on your child.

## Physical Health Concerns

Have you been using drugs, taking prescribed medications, or drinking alcohol that could affect the fetus?

Is it possible that this pregnancy is your last chance to have a child because of your age? Does your research suggest that the risk of birth defects increases after a specific age?

Are you physically well enough to carry a pregnancy to term without endangering yourself or your fetus? Are you well-nourished? Have you seen your gynecologist lately? If you were on a birth control pill when you got pregnant, let your gynecologist know, and discuss whether or not there may be any added risks of significance.

Do you have a medical illness (like lupus, congenital heart disease, diabetes) made worse by pregnancy? Did you have preeclampsia in your last pregnancy and become seriously ill? Did a doctor ever tell you that you should not get pregnant?

Is your pregnancy the result of sexual intercourse with someone in your own family, related to you genetically, that would increase your chance of having a child with birth defects or inheritable diseases?

Do you, or the biological father, have serious inheritable illnesses that may be transmitted to a child? If you are unsure, you could meet with a genetic counselor who can explain the odds of having a child with genetic deficits. As you become older, your overall risk of having a baby with birth defects rises. (See chapter 7, "Abortion Resources," for more information.) Have you looked at the risk for your particular age?

If you have a chronic illness, will that illness affect your ability to raise a child?

## Finances

Do you have school loans that will become due if you stop school?

Can you afford the cost of lost work and medical procedures associated with your pregnancy?

Can you afford to have a baby? You may want to look at "Single Motherhood Resources," chapter 5, and go to the BabyCenter.com website to determine how much it costs to have a baby.

If you are not working now, can you find a job that will support you and your child, given your job skills, education, and the economy? If you are working, is your job secure?

Does your job require working after hours, ability to travel on short notice, performing physically demanding work, being available on call, and flexibility that would be compromised by a baby/child/teenager's demands? Would your boss tolerate your missing work because of your child's illness? Will you be less productive if you're focusing on your child's needs?

How much will single parenthood impair your ability to find a new job if you need to, or if you find your job too burdensome?

Would you be willing to lower your standard of living and socioeconomic status? Would you be comfortable missing opportunities to meet men of your own class?

Can you make a living for you and your child at your current level of education?

Are you in good enough health to work, look after your baby, and do all the household chores and manage finances?

How will you afford financial emergencies like car repairs, moving expenses, and health crises?

Do you have enough cash reserves to manage if your job reduces your work time?

If you give birth to a special-needs child, will you be able to afford the added expenses and child care?

Will you be able to pay for child care?

## Your Energy

Will you be physically, mentally, and emotionally able to go home from work each day and start your second job of raising your child alone?

How do you plan to cope with often being tired and not getting enough sleep?

# A-3

*Supplementary Questions About Adoption*

The additional information and more detailed questions in this chapter may help clarify your thinking about adoption.

## Considering Different Perspectives

Could you find joy in knowing that, because of the adoption, somewhere a family has a child they longed for and a child has both a mother and father who are in a good position to raise the child? The four parents of your adoptive parents would be able to experience being grandparents as well.

Which of these statements is true? "A mother's chief goal is to make certain her child is raised the best possible way and has the best possible experience of life" or "A mother's chief goal is to make certain her child is raised the best way *she herself* can raise the child and has the best possible experience of life *she herself* can provide."

Would an adoptive mother supported financially by the adoptive father be in a better position to spend more time with their adopted child than a biological mother who must delegate responsibility to sitters, day care, and grandparents so she can work enough hours to provide for the child? Would an adoptive mother be less tired?

Are you considering raising the child because some of your

loved ones disapprove of adoption? Is this in the child's best interest?

## Explaining Your Adoption Process to Others

If you decide on adoption, at some point people will notice that you are no longer pregnant and don't have a child with you. Are you concerned about explaining your adoption decision to others? Is your belief that you've given your child a better life enough to help you deal with the questions you might get? Could you recruit your family's support in this?

## Selflessness

Do you think your child might one day realize that placing him or her with another family was the most loving, self-sacrificing thing that you could ever do? Even if your child initially might mistakenly believe you rejected him or her, do you think you could risk that anger because you believe that you're doing what's best?

Are you willing to experience being without your child, because you love him or her so much that you want the best for that child?

## The Adoptive Process

Are you aware that you can work with your adoption agency, your adoptive parents, and the hospital to individualize how your baby's transition to the adoptive parents happens?

Hospitals and agencies can provide opportunities for you to spend time with adoptive parents, have them with you while you are in the hospital, share the birth experience with them, and have a bonding experience with them that will help you feel better about trusting them with your child.

Hospitals and agencies can also work with you if you want to minimize all contact. Does having some control over this process make you less worried about panicking and changing your mind at the last minute?

Could your family help you put the adoption in a broader perspective, and help you with the grieving process? Could they remind you that you would probably be in a better position later to raise another child, and that your decision was not about whether you would have made a good mother?

Can you handle any remorse, feelings of failure, belief that you're not a good parent, or sense of feeling inferior that might interfere with your being able to pursue adoption?

Are you worried you will not be able to stop thinking whether you can trust your child to someone else's care? Will you think about someone else taking care of your child? Will you worry about what others will say, or obsess about what your child is doing?

If you have these particular concerns, you may want to talk with the adoption agency about an open adoption and maximizing your contact with your child. If you have an open adoption, how will you want to interact with the adoptive family?

## Added Responsibilities

For your baby to be healthy, you must see your OB/GYN doctor, eat healthy foods, take prenatal vitamins, avoid drinking, avoid smoking, and avoid using street drugs. It might require you to modify when and how you exercise, travel, or have sex. Do you have an OB/GYN who can help you with your health? An OB/GYN can be an important resource for you and will offer you his or her knowledge, experience, and emotional support.

## Anticipating Future Relationships

You may be worried that you and the adoptive mother will feel competitive, envious, or fearful toward each other. Do you realize that you may feel gratitude that she is trying her best to raise your child, and she may feel grateful to you for letting her? Do you think your common love for your child might permit you to have faith that you both have good intentions and later prevent your child from feeling as though his or her loyalty is torn between the two of you?

Can you plan how you will handle your relationship with the adopted child if you change partners or have more children?

How will you handle your adopted child wanting a relationship with his or her biological father?

# A-4

## Supplementary Questions About Abortion

The additional questions in this chapter may help clarify your thinking about abortion.

### Preconceived Ideas

Negative preconceived ideas about what kind of people have abortions may contribute to your having the baby when you do not want to. Unwanted motherhood has been shown to be destructive to the mother's mental health. Are your preconceived notions realistic? If you don't want a baby now, can you accept that?

### Another Abortion

If you had an abortion before, how is your situation different now?

If your situation is the same now as when you had your abortion, and you think you made the right decision, could it still be right for you to have an abortion now? Are there additional factors to consider now that weren't present then?

If your situation is the same now as when you had your abortion and you think you made the wrong decision then, do you feel that having a child now could undo it or make up for it? You cannot unring the bell. If it somehow could make up for it, is that reason enough to have a child? Is your decision in the best interest of the child, or made mainly from guilt about the earlier abortion?

## Rh Incompatibility

If you have Rh-negative blood, you will need to let your doctor know so he or she can give you Rh immunoglobulin to prevent you from becoming sensitized to your fetus's possible Rh-positive blood at the time of the abortion. It would also be important to tell your doctor about your being Rh negative if you have a miscarriage, because the same thing can happen at that time and you will need some immunoglobulin then as well.

# From the Author

Many people demonstrated their heartfelt caring about you by helping the author in the writing of this book. You have an opportunity to help other women now. When you are sure you are finished with this book, consider donating it.

Organizations would benefit from having this book to lend to women who might not otherwise discover it. These organizations include your local library, gynecologist's offices, family physician's offices, women's centers, college libraries, sororities, religious organizations, school counseling departments, and women's clinics. You may want to consider donating your book to a local agency that addresses the issues of family and children, or to agencies that promote education about family planning, single motherhood, adoption, or abortion.

You may not be experiencing an unplanned pregnancy yourself but have read this book for other reasons. You are in a position to help women by mentioning this book on social media like Facebook or Twitter.

Customer reviews make a big difference in how visible this book will be on Amazon. You can help other women find this book more easily by posting a review of it on Amazon. Let other women know why you found it useful. You don't need to write a long or formal review. A short summary of your thoughts would be very much appreciated. Thank you.

# Bibliography

The author does not endorse the content of these books or provide any sort of guarantee that they are accurate, timely, or complete.

Some of these books address topics that may be unrelated to your pregnancy but may help in understanding your life situation or the life situations of your family members.

*Adult Children of Alcoholics* by Janet Geringer Woititz

*A Lifelong Love Affair: Keeping Sexual Desire Alive in Your Relationship* by Joseph Nowinski

*Children of the Self-Absorbed: A Grown-Up's Guide to Getting Over Narcissistic Parents* by Nina W. Brown

*Choosing to Live: How to Defeat Suicide Through Cognitive Therapy* by Thomas Ellis and Cory Newman

*Codependent No More: How to Stop Controlling Others and Start Caring for Yourself* by Melody Beattie

*Emotional Blackmail: When the People in Your Life Use Fear, Obligation, and Guilt to Manipulate You* by Susan Forward and Donna Frazier

*Help Me Live: 20 Things People with Cancer Want You to Know* by Lori Hope

*In Good Conscience: A Practical, Emotional, and Spiritual*

*Guide to Deciding Whether to Have an Abortion* by Anna Runkle

*I Will Not Die an Unlived Life: Reclaiming Purpose and Passion* by Dawna Markova

*Making Peace with Your Parents* by Harold Bloomfield with Leonard Felder

*Pathfinders: Overcoming the Crises of Adult Life and Finding Your Own Path to Well-Being* by Gail Sheehy

*People of the Lie: The Hope for Healing Human Evil* by M. Scott Peck

*Pregnancy Options Workbook* by Margaret Johnston (Download it from http://www.pregnancyoptions.info)

*Reclaiming Your Life After Rape: Cognitive-Behavioral Therapy for Posttraumatic Stress Disorder Client Workbook (Treatments That Work)* by Barbara Olasov Rothbaum

*Reviving Ophelia: Saving the Selves of Adolescent Girls* by Mary Pipher and Ruth Ross

*Stronger Than Death: When Suicide Touches Your Life* by Sue Chance

*Taking the High Road: How to Cope with Your Ex-husband, Maintain Your Sanity, and Raise Your Child in Peace* by Nailah Shami

*Talking with Young Children About Adoption* by Mary Watkins and Susan Fisher

*The Complete Single Mother: Reassuring Answers to Your Most Challenging Concerns* by Andrea Engber and Leah Klungness

*The Hard Questions: 100 Questions to Ask Before You Say "I Do"* by Susan Piver

*The Script: The 100% Absolutely Predictable Things Men Do When They Cheat* by Elizabeth Landers and Vicki Mainzer

*The Single Mother's Survival Guide* by Patrice Karst

*Too Good to Leave, Too Bad to Stay: a Step-by-Step Guide to Help You Decide Whether to Stay in or Get Out of Your Relationship* by Mira Kirshenbaum

*Uncoupling: Turning Points in Intimate Relationships* by Diane Vaughn

*You Can Begin Again* by Gerald Mann

*You Can Read Anyone: Never Be Fooled, Lied to, or Taken Advantage of Again* by David J. Lieberman

*You Can't Say That to Me: Stopping the Pain of Verbal Abuse* by Suzette Haden Elgin

*When Bad Things Happen to Good People* by Harold S. Kushner

# Index

ABC Adoptions, 52
abortion
    avoidance-avoidance conflict, 24
    basic questions, 21–34
    the child's interests, 22, 25
    cost, 61
    D&C (dilation and curettage), 27
    D&E (dilation and evacuation), 31–32
    determining how far along you are, 56–57
    educating yourself, 55–56
    elective, 28–29
    emotional impact, 25–26, 62–64
    ethical issues, 21–24
    fetal pain issue, 62
    financial assistance, 60–61
    first-trimester, 58
    illegal, 26–28
    laws concerning, 6, 23, 29, 60, 64–65
    manual vacuum aspiration (MVA), 31, 58
    medical, 30, 57–58
    motherhood, lost chance of, 26
    negative preconceived ideas, 89
    pressure from others, 25
    pro-choice view, 22, 56
    pro-life view, 22
    providers, 59–60
    religious views, 23
    resources, 33–34, 55–66
    Rh incompatibility, 90
    risks, 20
    saline-induced, 32
    second, 89–90
    secret, 75
    spontaneous (miscarriage), 28, 90
    standard vacuum aspiration, 31–32, 58–59
    surgical, 30–32, 58–59
    timing of, 6, 24, 29, 32, 59
    types, 29–33
    waiting period, 60
    when life begins, 22–23
    where to get, 59–60
Abortion Care Network (ACN), 60
accredited colleges, 47–48

"Accuracy of Gestational Age Estimated by Menstrual Dating in Women Seeking Abortion Beyond Nine Weeks," 57

adoption
    adoptive parents, 17, 49, 53–54, 86–88
    advantages of two-parent families, 13–15
    basic questions, 13–20
    closed, 15
    expenses, 16–17
    explaining the process to others, 86
    foster home before, 15
    future relationship with your child, 17–18, 88
    by gay/lesbian couples, 14–15
    housing during pregnancy, 52–53
    how much say you have, 15
    husband's role/rights, 18
    independent, 51–52
    laws concerning, 52
    maternity homes, 52–53
    open, 15, 17, 50–51, 87
    perspectives on, 85–86
    private, 16
    process of, 86–87
    resources, 49–54
    responsibilities during pregnancy, 87
    risks in pregnancy/childbirth, 19–20
    scams, 54
    secret, 16–17, 19
    selflessness of, 86
    starting placement process early, 7
    teen pregnancy, 54
    types, 15–16

adoption agencies
    American Adoptions, 49–50
    contract with, 17
    Family Formation, 53
    finding, 51
    overview, 51
    Pact, 52
    the process, 86–87
    and your expenses, 16–17
    and your wishes, 15

Adoption.com, 53
Affordable Healthcare Act, 40
American Adoptions, 49–50
American College of Obstetricians and Gynecology, 54, 55
approach-approach conflict, 24
approach-avoidance conflict, 24
Arthur, Joyce: "Fetal Pain," 62
ASingleParents.com, 36
avoidance-avoidance conflict, 24

baby blues (postpartum depression), 45
BabyCenter.com, 36
BabyMed, 56
Backline, 55
bartering, 41
Before Abortion, 56
benefits.gov, 38

# Index

Big Brothers Big Sisters, 46
biological father
   and the adoption decision, 17–19
   child support from, 42
   determining, 56
   diseases inherited from, 76, 82
   ideal, 71
   life insurance for, 39–40
   other than husband, 76
   as parent material, 73
   parents of, 75–76
   passion to be a father, 72
   permanence in your life, 72
   personality, 73–74
   as a problem solver, 73
   protective vs. violent, 74–75
   as a provider, 73
   readiness of, 10, 72–73
   rights, 52
   and secret abortion or pregnancy, 75
   your relationship with, 71–72
birth control resources, 65–66
Boy Scouts, 46
Boys & Girls Clubs, 46
boys' relationship with fathers, 13–14

Caesarian section (C-section), 19–20
Centers for Disease Control and Prevention (CDC), 36
child support, 42
Child Welfare Information Gateway, 52
*Choosing to Live* (Ellis and Newman), 4, 45
cnpp.usda.gov, 36
CoAbode, 40
colleges, 47–48
*The Complete Single Mother* (Engber and Klungness), 35
conception calculator, 56
consumer.ftc.gov, 39
contraception resources, 65–66
credit cards, 41–42
credit counseling, 39

dating, 45–46
D&C (dilation and curettage), 27
D&E (dilation and evacuation), 31–32
the decision
   beliefs, reassuring, 3
   discussing with others, 2
   feelings underlying, 4
   the long view, 5
   making it yours, 1–2
   process of making, 6–7
   timing of, 6
   values underlying, 3
depression, 4
Division of Family and Children Services (DFACS), 50

education, 47–48
Ellis, Thomas: *Choosing to Live*, 4, 45

embryo, defined, 23
emotions. *See* feelings
Engber, Andrea: *The Complete Single Mother*, 35
Eunice Kennedy Shriver National Institute of Child Health and Human Development, 66

Family Formation, 53
family members. *See* parents
Family & Youth Services Bureau, 53
Feeding America, 39
feelings
    emotional impact of abortion, 25–26, 62–64
    ignoring vs. talking about them, 4
    self-destructive, 4
"Fetal Pain" (Arthur), 62
fetus
    defined, 23
    development, 55
    pain experienced during abortion, 62
    physical health concerns, 82
    ultrasound, 57
    viability, 23, 65
"50 Resources for Single Moms Going Back to College," 37
financial assistance, 38–39
food assistance, 38–39
gestation, defined, 29
gestational age, determining, 56–57
Girl Scouts, 46

girls' relationship with fathers, 14
God, reassuring beliefs about, 3
Goodwill, 40
grandparents reaction to unplanned pregnancy, 11
Guttmacher Institute, 65
gynecology, defined, 2

*The Hard Questions: 100 Questions to Ask Before You Say "I Do"* (Piver), 71
Health Center Searcher (Planned Parenthood), 60
health insurance, 40
husbands. *See also* biological father
    abusive/unstable, 18
    rights in adoption cases, 18
    unhappy marriage, 75
    vs. biological fathers, 76

immunoglobulin, 90
incest, 82
Independent Adoption Center (IAC), 51

job skills, 47–48
Johnston, Margaret: *Pregnancy Options Workbook*, 60

Karst, Patrice: *The Single Mother's Survival Guide*, 35
Kirshenbaum, Mira: *Too Good to Leave, Too Bad to Stay*, 71
Klungness, Leah: *The Complete Single Mother*, 35

legal fathers' rights, 18

Legal Match, 52

manual vacuum aspiration (MVA), 31, 58

maternity homes, 52–53

Medicaid, 40, 61

Medline Plus, 57, 58

Medscape, 58

mental health services, 45

mentoring programs, 46

methotrexate, 30

mifepristone (RU-486), 30

miscarriage (spontaneous abortion), 28, 90

misoprostol, 30

money management, 39–40

My Adoption Advisor, 54

National Abortion Federation (NAF), 58, 60–61, 62–63, 64

National Network of Abortion Funds, 61

National Suicide Hotline, 4, 45

Need Help Paying Bills, 38

needs vs. wants, 6

Newman, Cory: *Choosing to Live*, 4, 45

Northland Family Planning, 59

nutrition.gov, 43

OB/GYNs, 2, 87

obstetrics, defined, 2

One Harvest, 39

overload, avoiding, 3

Pact, 52

Parentbooks, 35

parenting skills, 5, 48, 79

parents
  adoptive, 17, 49, 53–54, 86–88
  of biological father, 75–76
  gay/lesbian, 14–15
  reaction to single motherhood, 11, 80–81
  reaction to unplanned pregnancy, 11

Parents.com, 36

Parents Without Partners, 37, 45

passivity, 7

Peer Resources, 46

Pell Grants, 47

perseverance, 7–8

pets, 41

Piver, Susan: *The Hard Questions: 100 Questions to Ask Before You Say "I Do"*, 71

placenta, 27

Planned Parenthood, 60, 61, 65

Planned Parenthood of Southeastern Virginia, 59

postpartum depression (baby blues), 45

preeclampsia, 19

pregnancy
  contraception resources, 65–66
  determining how far along you are, 56–57
  housing during, 52–53
  physical health concerns, 82

pregnancy, *continued*
   responsibilities during, 87
   risks, 19–20, 36
   teen, 54
Pregnancy Information Tool, 56
*Pregnancy Options Workbook* (Johnston), 60
Premier Diagnostic Services, 56
pride, 47
progesterone, 30

Rh incompatibility, 90
risks
   abortion, 20, 36
   pregnancy/childbirth, 19–20, 36
RU-486 (mifepristone), 30

scholarships, 47
sexual predators, 46
shyness, 47
single motherhood
   alternatives to having a child, 78
   approachability, 47
   avoiding extra expenses, 41–42
   avoiding paying full price, 41
   bartering, 41
   basic questions, 9–12
   books and book lists, 35–36
   child support, 42
   comprehensive websites, 37
   costs, 36
   dating, 45–46
   doing it yourself, 42
   education/job skills, 47–48
   effects on others, 80–81
   employment, 42–43, 83
   energy level, 84
   finances, 36, 39–40, 42–43, 83–84
   financial/food assistance, 38–39
   grants, 38–39, 47
   health insurance, 40
   helping your child get fathering, 46
   joys of, 77–78
   mental health services, 45
   money making, thinking creatively about, 42–43
   money management, 39–40
   perseverance needed, 7–8
   physical health concerns, 82
   questions about the biological father, 10
   questions about you, 9
   questions about your child, 10–11
   questions about your family, 11–12
   resources, 35–48
   risks of childbirth vs. abortion, 36
   saving money, 40
   sharing expenses, 40–41
   skills, 79
   and stress, 81
   taking care of yourself, 43–45
*The Single Mother's Survival Guide* (Karst), 35
singleparentsnetwork.com, 37

Special Supplemental Nutrition Program for Women, Infants, and Children (WIC), 39

"Sperm: How long do they live after ejaculation?" 56

spontaneous abortion (miscarriage), 28, 90

standard vacuum aspiration, 31–32, 58–59

Stotland, Nada Logan: "Abortion Trauma," 63

suicide hotline, 4, 45

Supplemental Nutrition Assistance Program (SNAP), 39

teen pregnancy, 54

Temporary Assistance for Needy Families (TANF), 38

TheBump.com, 55

*Too Good to Leave, Too Bad to Stay* (Kirshenbaum), 71

ultrasound, 57

values, 3

wants vs. needs, 6

WebMD, 58

WIC (Special Supplemental Nutrition Program for Women, Infants, and Children), 39

WomensHealth.gov, 65

YMCA and YWCA, 46

CPSIA information can be obtained at www.ICGtesting.com
Printed in the USA
LVOW10s0340190916

505088LV00001B/2/P